MRCS Core Modules: Practice Papers

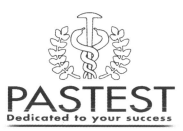

PASTEST
Dedicated to your success

MRCS Core Modules: Practice Papers

Christopher LH Chan
BSc (Hons) MB BS FRCS(Eng)
Sir Alan Parks and MRC Clinical Training Fellow

Academic Department of Surgery
St Bartholomew's and the Royal London
School of Medicine and Dentistry
Whitechapel, London
and
Specialist Registrar in General Surgery
South Thames (East) Rotation

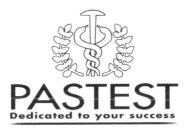

PASTEST
Dedicated to your success

© 2000 PASTEST
Egerton Court
Parkgate Estate
Knutsford
Cheshire
WA16 8DX

Telephone: 01565 752000

All rights reserved. No part of this publication may be reproduced, stored in a retrieval system, or transmitted, in any form or by any means, electronic, mechanical, photocopying, recording or otherwise without the prior permission of the copyright owner.

First published 2000
Reprinted 2001

ISBN: 1 901198 45 6

A catalogue record for this book is available from the British Library.

The information contained within this book was obtained by the authors from reliable sources. However, while every effort has been made to ensure its accuracy, no responsibility for loss, damage or injury occasioned to any person acting or refraining from action as a result of information contained herein can be accepted by the publishers or authors.

PasTest Revision Books and Intensive Courses

PasTest has been established in the field of postgraduate medical education since 1972, providing revision books and intensive study courses for doctors preparing for their professional examinations. Books and courses are available for the following specialties:
MRCS, MRCP Part 1 and 2, MRCPCH Part 1 and 2, MRCPsych, MRCOG, DRCOG, MRCGP, DCH, FRCA, PLAB.

For further details contact:

PasTest, Freepost, Knutsford, Cheshire WA16 7BR
Tel: 01565 752000   Fax: 01565 650264

Text prepared by Breeze Ltd, Manchester.
Printed and bound by Ashford Colour Press, Gosport, Hants.

CONTENTS

CONTRIBUTORS

Mr Sam Andrews MA MS FRCS
Consultant General and Vascular Surgeon, Maidstone and Tunbridge Wells NHS Trust, Maidstone General Hospital, Maidstone, Kent.

Professor Martin Berry MD DSc FRCPath
Professor of Anatomy, Centre for Neuroscience, Neural Damage and Repair, Hodgkin Building, Guy's Campus, London.

Mr John Bowen FRCS (Paed)
Consultant Neonatal and Paediatric Surgeon, Department of Paediatric Surgery, Royal Manchester Children's Hospital, Pendlebury, Manchester.

Mr Christopher LH Chan Bsc(Hons) MBBS FRCS(Eng)
Sir Alan Parks and MRC Clinical Training Fellow, Academic Department of Surgery, St Bartholomew's and the Royal London School of Medicine and Dentistry, Whitechapel, London and Specialist Registrar in General Surgery, South Thames (East) Rotation

Miss Shirley Chan FRCS
Higher Surgical Trainee, Conquest Hospital, St. Leonards on Sea, East Sussex.

Mr Matthew Dunn FRCS FFAEM DIMC DSMRSC
Consultant in Accident and Emergency, Department of Accident and Emergency, Warwick Hospital, Warwick.

Ms Deborah Eastwood MB FRCS
Consultant Orthopaedic Surgeon, (Honorary Senior Lecturer), Paediatric Unit, Royal National Orthopaedic Hospital, Brockley Hill, Stanmore, Middlesex.

Mr Jeremy J Elkabir MBBS FRCS (Eng) FRCS Urol
Senior Registrar in Urology, St George's Hospital, London.

Mr Andrew J Malouf MBBS (Syd) FRACS
Locum Consultant Colorectal Surgeon, Department of Colorectal Surgery, St Mark's Hospital, Watford Road, Harrow, London and Central Middlesex Hospital, Park Royal, London.

Dr Terry Martin MSc MB BS DRCOG DavMed MRCS DIMC RCSEd Associate Fellow FAEM
Specialist Registrar in Anaesthetics, Nuffield Department of Anaesthetics, John Radcliffe Hospital, Oxford.

Mr Charles Maxwell-Armstrong DM FRCS
Specialist Registrar in General Surgery, Department of Surgery, Queen's Medical Centre, Nottingham.

Mr John Mosley BSc MD MRCP FRCS (England and Edinburgh)
Consultant General Surgeon, Leigh Infirmary, Leigh, Lancashire.

Dr Andrew Mumford BSc MB ChB MRCP
Research Fellow, MRC Haemostasis Research Group, Clinical Sciences Centre, Hammersmith Hospital, London.

Dr R E Shanthakumar MB BS FFARCSI FRCA EDICM
Consultant Anaesthetist, Department of Anaesthetics, Barnet General Hospital, Barnet, Herts.

Dr David Southern FRCA
Consultant Anaesthetist, Department of Anaesthesia, Wrexham Maelor Hospital, Wrexham, North Wales.

PREFACE

This book is intended primarily for candidates sitting the Core MCQ section of the MRCS/AFRCS examination. The papers have been specifically structured as Practice papers and aim to reflect the Royal College Syllabus.

The goal of such a book is to provide an adjunct to reading, help assess knowledge and alert one to areas that require further study. In addition, this book has covered the favourite topics that appear in the MRCS/AFRCS examinations. MCQ practice will increase basic knowledge and detailed explanations have been written to aid revision. The explanations should also be useful to candidates in other parts of the examination.

I hope that this book will not be restricted only to candidates sitting the MRCS/AFRCS examination but will also be of use to Final Year medical students.

Christopher Chan
August 2000

INTRODUCTION

In 1997 the structure of the surgical diploma examinations underwent a series of major changes, in which the 'old-style FRCS' exam was replaced by the new 'entry-level' qualifications of the MRCS (MRCSEd, MRCS (Glasg.) or AFRCSI). A pass is required in all sections of the MRCS Diploma Examination, which is taken during approved basic surgical training (24 month period). Having completed the MRCS, the trainee can then apply for a national training number (NTN) and commence higher surgical training in his or her chosen surgical specialty. A final exit examination is then required in that specialty. A pass in the Intercollegiate specialty examination awards the candidate with the 'full' Fellowship of the Royal College of Surgeons (FRCS). Providing training has been adequately completed, the trainee can then apply for a certificate of completion of Surgical Training (CCST) and be placed on the GMC register and so be eligible to apply for a consultant post.

Membership of the Royal College of Surgeons of England (MRCS) examination consists of three sections:

1. Two multiple choice papers: (conducted twice a year)
        Paper 1 - Core Modules (2 hrs duration)
        Paper 2 - System Modules (2 hrs duration)
2. A Clinical Section (conducted twice a year)
3. A Viva Voce section (conducted twice a year)

The first section consists of two multiple choice papers.
Paper 1 Core Modules tests knowledge of peri-operative management, trauma, intensive care, neoplasia, techniques and outcomes of surgery.
Paper 2 System Modules involves specific systems: locomotor, vascular, abdominal, head, neck, endocrine and paediatric, urology and renal transplantation. These subjects are tested using a combination of multiple choice questions and extended matching questions.

Candidates may sit each of the MCQ papers as often as they wish.

The format for the AFRCS offered by the Royal College of Surgeons in Edinburgh is almost identical to the MRCS, and consists of two multiple choice exams – Principles of Surgery in General and Systematic Surgery. Both papers can be taken at any time during the two years of basic surgical training. The Royal College of Surgeons in Glasgow contain four

1-hour MCQ question papers covering: anatomy, physiology, pathology and clinical surgery. These papers can be taken after a minimum of 9 months of basic surgical training. The MCQ papers are all held on the same day. The Royal College of Surgeons in Ireland has three parts. There are four 1-hour papers, each containing 20 questions on: surgical anatomy, surgical physiology, applied pathology, microbiology, immunology and clinical surgery. There is full reciprocity of recognition of a 'pass' in the whole MCQ section between all three UK Royal Surgical Colleges and the Royal College of Surgeons of Ireland.

The candidate then progresses to the Clinical and Viva sections of the exam. For the Royal College of Surgeons of England MRCS exam, a candidate must pass the written papers before sitting the clinical examination, and pass both written and clinical before being invited to the Viva. In other colleges the order varies slightly. Only when a candidate has passed all three parts of the examination are they awarded the MRCS Diploma.

MCQ EXAMINATION TECHNIQUE

Exam technique

Before sitting an MCQ examination, you will need to know how many questions are likely to be on the paper and how long you will be given to complete it. Thus you will be able to assess the approximate amount of time that can be spent on each question. The time allotted for each of the written papers is **two hours**. Different questions are used each time, therefore subject composition is variable from exam to exam. There are approximately 45 MCQs and around 20 EMQs, depending upon the number of responses required.

Pacing yourself accurately during the examination to finish on time, or with time to spare, is essential. You must also decide on your own personal strategy for approaching the paper. You may decide to read quickly through the paper before picking up your pen, or to work slowly through the paper answering everything that you are certain of and leaving anything you wish to come back to.

There are two common mistakes which cause good candidates to fail the MRCS written examinations. These are neglecting to read the directions and questions carefully enough and failing to fill in the computer answer card properly. You must read the instructions to candidates at the beginning of each section of the paper to ensure that you complete the answer sheet correctly. You must also ensure that you read the question (both stem and items) carefully. Regard each item as being independent of every other item, each referring to a specific quantum of knowledge. The item (or the stem and the item taken together) make up a statement as 'True' or 'False'. The number of stems will vary for each question. For this reason, a mark will not necessarily be required for each column of the answer sheet. For every correct answer you will gain a mark (+1). For the MRCS (London) examination, marks will not be deducted for a wrong answer. Equally, you will not gain a mark if you mark both true and false.

You must also decide on a strategy to follow with regard to marking your answers. The answer sheet is read by an automatic document reader, which transfers the information it reads to a computer. It is critical that the answer sheet is filled in clearly and accurately using the pencils provided. Failure to fill in your name and your examination correctly could result in the rejection of your paper. Some candidates mark their answers directly onto the computer sheet as they go through the question, others prefer to make a note of their answers on the question paper, and reserve time at the end to transfer their answers onto the computer sheet. If you choose the first method, there is a chance that you may decide to change your answer after a second reading. If you do change your answer on the computer sheet, you must ensure that your original is thoroughly erased. If you choose the second method, make sure that you allow enough time to transfer your answers methodically onto the computer sheet, as rushing at this stage could introduce some costly mistakes. You will find it less confusing if you transfer your marks after you have completed each section of the examination. You must ensure that you have left sufficient time to transfer your marks from the question paper to the answer sheet. You should also be aware that no additional time will be given at the end of the examination to allow you to transfer your marks.

If you find that you have time left at the end of the examination, there can be a temptation to re-read your answers time and time again, so that even those that seemed straightforward will start to look less convincing. In this situation, first thoughts are usually the best, don't alter your initial answers unless you are sure. Don't be afraid to leave the examination room once you are satisfied with your answers.

To guess or not to guess

Tests carried out at PasTest's MRCS intensive revision courses have proved that most candidates can improve their marks by making sensible guesses.

The MRCS exams in England are not negatively marked[1]. For this reason you should answer every question as you have nothing to lose. If you do not know the answer to a question, you should make an educated guess – you may well get the answer right and gain a mark.

If you feel that you need to spend more time puzzling over a question, leave it and, if you have time, return to it. Make sure you have collected all the marks you can before you come back to any difficult questions.

Final advice

Multiple choice questions are not designed to trick you or confuse you, they are designed to test your knowledge of surgery. Accept each question at its face value, do not look for hidden meanings or catches. The aim of this book is to enable you to evaluate your level of knowledge by working through the questions in each section. By marking clearly all of the answers that you got wrong or declined to answer, you can then refresh your memory with the explanations given here or read up on specific topics in depth using a textbook.

Working through the questions in this book will help you to identify your weak subject areas. Using books and lectures, you must work out your own personal profile of strengths and weaknesses and plan your revision accordingly. In the last few weeks before the exam it will be important for you to avoid minor unimportant areas and concentrate on the most important subject areas covered in the exam.

---

[1] The AFRCS examinations in Scotland are currently negatively marked. (Jun 2001)

SAMPLE MCQ ANSWER SHEET

THE ROYAL COLLEGE OF SURGEONS OF ENGLAND

MRCS

1

This document is designed to be machine readable.
Please use the pencil provided.
If you make a mistake please use an eraser.
Mark for True.
Mark for False.
Candidates are reminded that a standard answer sheet is being used!
The number of items will vary for each question, therefore, a mark will not
necessarily be required for each column of the answer sheet.

For example,
candidate 0076 should
be inserted as:

Candidate Number

Please insert your
candidate number
as shown above.

Sample answer sheet, reproduced by kind permission of
the Royal College of Surgeons of England

SAMPLE EMQ ANSWER SHEET

Each question will have up to ten options listed (A–J). Only one of the options will be the correct answer. Indicate your response by marking a single line through the appropriate box.

For example:
Question 61 correct answer is option C
Question 62 correct answer is option F
Question 63 correct answer is option A

Sample answer sheet, reproduced by kind permission of the Royal College of Surgeons of England

GLOSSARY

5-FU	5-fluorouracil
AAA	Abdominal aortic aneurysm
ACTH	Adrenocorticotropic hormone
ADH	Anti-diuretic hormone
ANOVA	Analysis of variance
ANP	Atrial natriuretic peptide
AP	Antero-posterior
APTT	Activated partial thromboplastin time
ARDS	Adult respiratory distress syndrome
ARF	Acute renal failure
AXR	Abdominal X-ray
BCC	Basal cell carcinoma
BPH	Benign prostatic hyperplasia
CEA	Carcinoembryonic antigen
CPAP	Continuous positive airway pressure
CPP	Central perfusion pressure
CPR	Cardio-pulmonary resuscitation
CRP	C-reactive protein
CSF	Cerebrospinal fluid
CT	Computerised tomography
CVP	Central venous pressure
CXR	Chest X-ray
DCIS	Ductal carcinoma in situ
DES	Diethylstilbestrol
DIC	Disseminated intravascular coagulation
DMSA	Dimercaptosuccinic acid
DPL	Diagnostic peritoneal lavage
DTPA	Diethylene triamine penta-acetic
ECG	Electrocardiograph
ERC	European resuscitation council
ERCP	Endoscopic retrograde cholangiopancreatography
ESR	Erythrocyte sedimentation rate
ESWL	Extra-corporeal shock wave lithotripsy
EUA	Examination under anaesthetic
FAP	Familial adenomatous polyposis
FBC	Full blood count
FFAs	Free fatty acids
FFP	Fresh frozen plasma
FIB	Fibrinogen
FNAC	Fine needle aspiration cytology
FOBT	Faecal occult blood testing
FRC	Functional residual capacity
GCS	Glasgow Coma Scale

GFR	Glomerular filtration rate
GI	Gastrointestinal
GTN	Glyceryl trinitrate
GVHD	Graft versus host disease
HIFU	High intensity focused ultrasound
HNPCC	Hereditary non-polyposis colorectal cancer
IBD	Inflammatory bowel disease
ICP	Intracranial pressure
IDDM	Insulin dependent diabetes mellitus
INR	International normalised ratio
ITGCN	Intra-tubular germ cell neoplasia
IVU	Intravenous urogram
KUB	Kidneys, ureter, bladder
LMWH	Low molecular weight heparins
MAOIs	Monoamine oxidase inhibitors
MAP	Mean arterial blood pressure
MEN	Multiple endocrine neoplasia
MIBG scan	Meta-iodobenzyl guanidine
MODS	Multiple organ dysfunction syndrome
MRA	Magnetic resonance angiography
MRSA	Methicillin-resistant Staphylococcus aureus
MSU	Midstream urine
NEC	Necrotising enterocolitis
NSAID	Non-steroidal anti-inflammatory drugs
OA	Oesophageal atresia
PCNL	Percutaneous nephrolithotomy
PEEP	Positive end expiratory pressure
PMC	Pseudomembranous colitis
PSA	Prostatic specific antigen
PT	Prothrombin time
PUJ	Pelvi-ureteric junction
RBC	Red blood cells
RCC	Renal cell carcinoma
RTA	Road traffic accident
SCC	Squamous cell carcinoma
SSG	Split skin grafting
TIA	Transient ischaemic attack
TOF	Tracheo-oesophageal fistula
TPN	Total parenteral nutrition
TRUS	Transrectal ultrasound scan
TT	Thrombin time
TURBT	Trans-urethral resection of bladder tumour
TURP	Transurethral resection of the prostate
UDT	Undescended testis
UTI	Urinary Tract Infection
vWF	von Willebrand factor
WBC	White blood cells

Time allowed: 2 hours
Indicate your answers in the spaces provided

CORE PAPER 1
SECTION 1 – MCQS

1. **Concerning wound healing**

    ❑ A most skin wounds regain their pre-injury strength with time
    ❑ B wound strength returns to 80% of pre-injury strength by three months (uncomplicated cases)
    ❑ C the small bowel regains most of its strength by ten days
    ❑ D type III collagen is stronger than type I collagen
    ❑ E skin healing includes a lag phase lasting six weeks following injury

2. **Metabolic responses to surgery include**

    ❑ A increased aldosterone secretion
    ❑ B reduced growth hormone secretion
    ❑ C reduced catecholamine secretion
    ❑ D increased thyroxine secretion
    ❑ E increased ADH secretion

3. **Antibiotic prophylaxis in surgery**

    ❑ A iv antibiotics given three hours following a right hemicolectomy are effective in preventing infection
    ❑ B some degree of contamination occurs in all operations
    ❑ C with the exception of prolonged operations, single dose prophylaxis is effective in most clinical situations
    ❑ D prophylaxis should be used wherever the risk of wound infection is increased
    ❑ E choice of the antibiotic antimicrobial spectrum is not important

4. **Oesophageal cancer**

☐ A has an overall 5-year survival of less than 10%
☐ B has an overall 1-year survival of about 75%
☐ C is associated with prominent lymphatic permeation
☐ D is associated with β naphthylamine exposure
☐ E stenting is a valuable palliative option for upper-third tumours

5. **Radiotherapy for breast cancer**

☐ A has been clearly shown to improve overall survival
☐ B has been clearly shown to reduce local recurrence rates
       following conservative breast surgery
☐ C should be applied to the axilla, if axillary clearance reveals
       three or more involved lymph nodes
☐ D is the treatment of choice for the palliation of painful bone
       metastases
☐ E generally includes an extra boost to the internal mammary
       chain lymph nodes for lateral tumours

6. **Regarding local surgery for breast cancer, which of the
    following are relative indications for conservative breast
    excision rather than mastectomy**

☐ A small tumours
☐ B oestrogen receptor positivity
☐ C impalpable disease
☐ D menopausal status
☐ E patient choice

7. **Regarding bone tumours**

☐ A malignant primary bone tumours are rare
☐ B the commonest bone tumour is a metastasis from a primary
       malignant tumour at another site
☐ C Ewing's sarcoma has a good prognosis
☐ D benign bone tumours tend to occur in the elderly
☐ E primary malignant bone tumours usually run an indolent
       clinical course

8. **Risk factors for male breast carcinoma include**

❏ A family history
❏ B smoking
❏ C testosterone antagonists
❏ D Klinefelter's syndrome
❏ E orchidectomy

9. **Characteristic features of HNPCC (hereditary non-polyposis colorectal cancer) include**

❏ A late age of onset of colorectal cancer
❏ B an increased incidence of proximal bowel cancer compared to the general population
❏ C an increased incidence of endometrial cancer compared to the general population
❏ D a worse 5-year survival compared to colonic carcinoma in the general population
❏ E a low incidence of mucinous carcinomas compared to colonic carcinomas in the general population

10. **Interpretation of the results of screening programmes for cancer must allow for the following types of bias:**

❏ A selection bias
❏ B calculation bias
❏ C detection bias
❏ D length bias
❏ E lead-time bias

11. **Third space fluid loss in the peri-operative period**

❏ A is related to degree of tissue injury
❏ B can be up to 15 ml/kg/hr
❏ C has fluid composition similar to interstitial fluid
❏ D is best replaced by dextrose saline
❏ E includes losses from entero-cutaneous fistulae

12. **Complications of epidural anaesthetic include**

- A post-dural puncture headache
- B hypertension
- C bradycardia
- D urine retention
- E hyperventilation

13. **A preparation of 10 ml of 0.5% bupivacaine heavy with 1 in 200,000 adrenaline**

- A is isobaric
- B contains 5 mg of bupivacaine
- C contains 500 µg of adrenaline
- D contains 8% dextrose
- E is suitable for intravenous injection

14. **Dopexamine**

- A has α-adrenergic actions even at low dose
- B has a natriuretic action
- C has little effect on the mean arterial pressure
- D increases the cardiac index by reducing systemic vascular resistance
- E is nephrotoxic

15. **A 50-year-old man with Type I diabetes mellitus is scheduled for elective cholecystectomy**

- A pre-operative investigations should include U&E, FBC, CXR and ECG
- B the best assessment of his normal diabetic control is random blood glucose
- C should not receive insulin on the morning of surgery in case he becomes hypoglycaemic
- D all blood glucose tests should be sent to the laboratory as bedside tests are too inaccurate
- E the Alberti regimen may be applicable

4

16.   **Multiple organ dysfunction syndrome (MODS)**

❏   A   outcome is improved by the use of pulmonary artery catheters
❏   B   only occurs after major trauma
❏   C   may involve inflammatory mediators
❏   D   when treated aggressively has a universally excellent outcome
❏   E   survival is increased with administration of endotoxin
            antibodies

17.   **The oxygen haemoglobin dissociation curve is displaced to
the left by**

❏   A   increase in pH
❏   B   anaemia
❏   C   fall in pCO_2
❏   D   pyrexia
❏   E   fall in 2,3 DPG

18.   **Angiotensin II**

❏   A   stimulates renin release
❏   B   inhibits aldosterone release
❏   C   is a weak arteriolar vasoconstrictor
❏   D   is converted from angiotensin I in the lung
❏   E   is released by hypovolaemia

19.   **Baseline investigations for a patient with major burns include**

❏   A   glycosylated haemoglobin
❏   B   arterial blood gases
❏   C   CXR
❏   D   AXR
❏   E   thoracic CT

20. **With regards to fluid replacement for bleeding secondary to trauma**

❏ A   excessive crystalloid administration may lead to the development of adult respiratory distress syndrome (ARDS)
❏ B   initial volume expansion is more quickly achieved with crystalloid rather than colloid
❏ C   colloid administration prevents a fall in haematocrit level
❏ D   stored blood has a high pH
❏ E   blood is the fluid of choice to replace ongoing haemorrhage and hypotension

21. **During management of a multi-traumatised patient**

❏ A   primary and secondary surveys should be repeated frequently to ascertain deterioration in patient status
❏ B   penile meatal blood is a contraindication to urethral catheterisation
❏ C   gastric tubes should not be passed trans-nasally if there is suspicion of a cribriform plate fracture
❏ D   skull X-rays are valuable in making immediate management decisions
❏ E   blood pressure is a good measure of actual tissue perfusion

22. **In pelvic trauma**

❏ A   mechanically unstable pelvic injuries involve at least two disruptions of the ring
❏ B   blood loss is best controlled by mechanical stabilisation of the pelvis
❏ C   acetabular fractures are usually difficult to see on AP X-rays of the pelvis
❏ D   acetabular fractures are caused by anterior pressure on the pubic rami

23. **Traumatic rupture of the thoracic aorta**

☐ A usually occurs just distal to the origin of the left subclavian artery
☐ B is most common following an acceleration injury
☐ C may cause a widened upper mediastinum and tracheal displacement
☐ D is best demonstrated by CT scan
☐ E is usually fatal

24. **Partial thickness burns**

☐ A commonly result from contact with hot fluids
☐ B have a pale or white appearance
☐ C have a weeping surface
☐ D are painless and insensitive
☐ E are sensitive to air

25. **Tissue hypoxia caused by chest trauma results from**

☐ A pulmonary ventilation-perfusion mismatch
☐ B hypocarbia
☐ C hypovolaemia
☐ D changes in the intra-thoracic pressure relationships
☐ E alveolar hypersensitivity

26. **The Glasgow Coma Scale incorporates details on**

☐ A the best verbal response to stimulation
☐ B peripheral reflex activity
☐ C systolic blood pressure on arrival in the A&E Department
☐ D pulse rate following initial resuscitation
☐ E eye opening to stimulation

27.   **Signs of pulmonary thromboembolism may include**

❏   A   ECG pattern of $S_1Q_3T_3$
❏   B   elevated arterial pCO_2
❏   C   mismatched defects on ventilation-perfusion lung scan
❏   D   pleural effusion on CXR
❏   E   obstruction to the pulmonary circulation on pulmonary angiography

28.   **The following can be measured (directly or indirectly) using Swan-Ganz catheterisation:**

❏   A   cardiac index
❏   B FiO_2
❏   C   left ventricular stroke work
❏   D   end tidal CO_2
❏   E   pulmonary artery occlusion pressure

29.   **Concerning cutaneous naevi**

❏   A   junctional activity is a prominent feature of intra-dermal naevi
❏   B   junctional naevi have a high malignant potential
❏   C   compound naevi have both junctional activity and intra-dermal components
❏   D   halo naevi have a predilection to infiltrate nerves

30.   **Rectal anastomosis**

❏   A   below the peritoneal reflection has a higher leak rate compared with those above
❏   B   fashioned by the double-layered technique is superior to the single-layered technique
❏   C   using staples has a significantly lower clinical leak rate than a handsewn anastomosis
❏   D   has a higher radiological than clinical leak rate
❏   E   fashioned using non-absorbable suture materials give superior functional results

31. **Concerning viral hepatitis**

❑ A persistence of hepatitis B sAg indicates an increased risk of developing chronic liver disease
❑ B chronic hepatitis B infection increases the risk of developing gall bladder carcinoma
❑ C hepatitis C virus accounts for about 90% of post-transfusion hepatitis
❑ D the acute illness of hepatitis C virus is generally less severe than that of hepatitis B virus

32. **Actinomycosis infection**

❑ A is very sensitive to penicillin treatment
❑ B is frequently found in association with other bacteria
❑ C is produced by Gram-negative rods
❑ D may mimic inflammatory bowel disease
❑ E usually resolves with antibiotics when associated with abscess formation

33. *Clostridium difficile*

❑ A infection has been increasing in incidence in the past ten years
❑ B infection is only caused by antibiotic treatment
❑ C infection is most commonly caused by gentamicin
❑ D induced diarrhoea typically starts within a week of commencing antibiotics
❑ E spores may be found in dust

34. **An enlarging pituitary gland may cause**

❑ A an homonymous hemianopia
❑ B depression of the pupillary reflexes
❑ C blockage of drainage from the cavernous dural venous sinus
❑ D erosion of the posterior ethmoid air sinuses
❑ E erosion of the anterior clinoid processes

35. **After an upper C7 spinal cord hemi-transection there is ipsilateral**

   ❑ A   loss of pain sensation in the axilla
   ❑ B   brisk biceps tendon reflex
   ❑ C   wasting of the thenar eminence
   ❑ D   claw hand
   ❑ E   winged scapula

36. **The thoracic duct**

   ❑ A   lies on the posterior intercostal vessels
   ❑ B   has no valves
   ❑ C   runs through the thoracic inlet to the left of the oesophagus
   ❑ D   receives the right bronchomediastinal lymph trunk
   ❑ E   arches over the left suprapleural membrane

37. **The hilum of the left lung**

   ❑ A   has the phrenic nerve lying anterior
   ❑ B   has the vagus nerve lying posterior
   ❑ C   contains upper and lower lobe bronchi
   ❑ D   is separated from the aortic arch by the vagus nerve
   ❑ E   has the pulmonary artery anterior to the main bronchus

38. **The aortic arch**

   ❑ A   lies anterior to the brachiocephalic veins
   ❑ B   gives attachment to the pre-tracheal fascia
   ❑ C   arches directly over the right pulmonary artery
   ❑ D   arches above the manubriosternal joint
   ❑ E   is covered by pleura

39.   **Intervertebral disc collapse between L5 and S1**

☐   A   would crush the L5 spinal nerve
☐   B   would impinge into the sacral segments of the cord
☐   C   usually causes pain to radiate over the medial malleolus
☐   D   would exaggerate the tendon reflex at the ankle
☐   E   may cause reduced sweating over the posterior aspect of the calf

40.   **Prolongation of the activated partial thromboplastin time (APTT)**

☐   A   usually occurs with low molecular weight heparin treatment
☐   B   occurs after warfarin treatment
☐   C   indicates adequacy of thrombo-prophylaxis with subcutaneous heparin
☐   D   is usual in patients receiving intravenous heparin
☐   E   may indicate a lupus anticoagulant

41.   **In haemophilia**

☐   A   mucosal membrane bleeding is the hallmark of haemophilia A
☐   B   female carriers of haemophilia A have no bleeding tendency
☐   C   haemophilia B is inherited as an autosomal recessive trait
☐   D   haemophilia B is a deficiency in factor IX
☐   E   pseudotumours may complicate intra-muscular bleeds in haemophilia A

42.   **Fresh frozen plasma**

☐   A   must be thawed on the ward or in the operating theatre
☐   B   contains albumin
☐   C   may cause a severe transfusion reaction
☐   D   contains immunoglobulins
☐   E   is the blood product of choice for replacing fibrinogen

43. **In the pre-operative correction of coagulation defects**

- ❏ A fresh frozen plasma may be used to correct the clotting defect in liver disease
- ❏ B a PT of less than 18 s requires correction before abdominal surgery
- ❏ C cryoprecipitate is useful if the APTT is greater than 55 s
- ❏ D fresh frozen plasma should be given as close to surgery as possible
- ❏ E fresh frozen plasma is the treatment of choice in haemophilia A

44. **Red cell units for transfusion**

- ❏ A have a shelf life of four days
- ❏ B must be transfused within five hours of leaving controlled storage
- ❏ C must be ABO and rhesus D identical to the recipient
- ❏ D have a volume of approximately 280 ml per unit
- ❏ E have a decreasing concentration of extracellular potassium with age

45. **Acute haemolytic transfusion reactions**

- ❏ A are most severe if group O cells are transfused into a group A recipient
- ❏ B may present with loin pain
- ❏ C are usually due to ABO typing errors
- ❏ D may cause haemoglobinuria
- ❏ E are clinically similar to the effects of bacterially contaminated blood

46. In statistical analysis

❑ A a Type I error is finding results that are not statistically significant when the populations are identical

❑ B a Type II error is finding a statistically significant result when the populations are identical

❑ C an unpaired t-test compares two groups on the assumption that the two populations are normally distributed

❑ D parametric tests are used when data from population groups do not follow a Gaussian distribution

❑ E non-parametric tests are less powerful than parametric tests

47. Clinical audit in surgical practice

❑ A needs to be surgeon led

❑ B assesses an endpoint associated with a particular clinical intervention

❑ C may include altering clinical practice if findings suggest improvements can be made

❑ D must include detailed clinical information on patients

❑ E is more reliable if data collection is carried out prospectively

Theme: Microbiology following skin trauma

A   *Staphylococcus aureus*
B   *Streptococcus pyogenes*
C   *Pasteurella multocida*
D   *Streptococcus milleri*
E   *Pseudomonas aeruginosa*

For each of the clinical scenarios listed below, select the most likely offending pathogen from the list of organisms above. Each option may be used once, more than once, or not at all.

- [ ] 61. Carbuncles
- [ ] 62. Infected dog bites
- [ ] 63. Cellulitis
- [ ] 64. Styes
- [ ] 65. Infected human bites
- [ ] 66. Infected leg ulcers

Theme: Wounds

A   Sterile
B   Clean
C   Clean-contaminated
D   Contaminated
E   Indeterminate

For each of the clinical scenarios listed below, select the most likely classification of wound from the list above. Each option may be used once, more than once, or not at all.

- [ ] 67. The small bowel has been entered but without significant spillage of contents
- [ ] 68. A non-infected biliary tract has been entered
- [ ] 69. Crush wound to the leg
- [ ] 70. An infected genito-urinary tract has been entered
- [ ] 71. Scalpel incision for a ganglion excision
- [ ] 72. Inadvertent incision into the vagina

Theme: Burns in children

A   1%
B   4.5%
C   7%
D   9%
E   14%
F   18%

For each of the clinical scenarios regarding cutaneous burns in children listed below, select the most likely percentage of the total body surface area from the list above. Each option may be used once, more than once, or not at all.

☐   73.   Burns to all the head and neck
☐   74.   Burns to all the anterior trunk (chest and abdomen)
☐   75.   Burns to all the male genitalia
☐   76.   Burns to all the posterior trunk (upper and lower back)
☐   77.   Burns to the whole anterior aspect of one leg
☐   78.   Burns to the whole aspect of one arm
☐   79.   Burns to the posterior aspect of both legs

Theme: Hormone secreting tumours

A   Calcitonin
B   Erythropoietin
C   5 hydroxytryptamine
D   Growth hormone
E   α–fetoprotein
F   ACTH

For each of the tumours listed below, select the most likely hormone produced by the tumour from the list above. Each option may be used once, more than once, or not at all.

☐   80.   Testicular teratoma
☐   81.   Bronchial carcinoma
☐   82.   Medullary thyroid carcinoma
☐   83.   Carcinoid tumour
☐   84.   Hypernephroma
☐   85.   Pituitary adenoma

Theme: Paraneoplastic syndromes

A   Multiple myeloma
B   Pancreatic carcinoma
C   Colon carcinoma
D   Renal carcinoma
E   Thymoma
F   Lymphoma

For each of the clinical systemic manifestations below, select the tumour most likely to produce these effects from the list above. Each option may be used once, more than once, or not at all.

☐   86.   Myasthenia gravis
☐   87.   Polycythaemia
☐   88.   Hypercalcaemia
☐   89.   Hyperglycaemia

Theme: Peripheral nerve anatomy

A   Facial nerve
B   Lingual nerve
C   Ophthalmic nerve
D   Trochlear nerve
E   Cranial accessory nerve
F   Oculomotor nerve
G   Glossopharyngeal nerve
H   Cervical sympathetic trunk

For each of the patients below, select the nerve most likely to be involved from the list above. Each option may be used once, more than once or not at all.

☐   90.   Two days after a left lower wisdom tooth extraction, a fit 23-year-old man complains of a severe bleed from the left side of his tongue, which he has bitten. The tongue is insensitive to touch and taste stimuli on the left.
☐   91.   A fit 26-year-old man suddenly develops a persistent dry left eye, clouded vision, blunted taste sensation, and an inability to empty food from the left vestibule.
☐   92.   A 25-year-old woman develops a left-sided ptosis and a dilated pupil.

❑ 93. A 25 year-old woman develops a left-sided ptosis and a constricted pupil.

❑ 94. A 40-year-old woman complains of clouding vision in the left eye after development of a rash over the left side of the forehead. She has burning pain over the left forehead and in the left eye, but no ptosis or diplopia. The corneal reflex is intact.

Theme: Structures in the transthoracic plane (of Louis)

A   Trachea
B   Superior vena cava
C   Mediastinal parietal pleura
D   T4 vertebra
E   Left brachiocephalic vein
F   Left pulmonary artery
G   Vagus nerve
H   2nd costal cartilage
I   Ascending aorta
J   Thoracic duct
K   Oesophagus
L   Left main bronchus

For each of the statements below, select the most likely option from the list above. Each option may be used once, more than once or not at all.

❑ 95. Gives off a branch which ascends between the trachea and oesophagus
❑ 96. Gives attachment to pre-vertebral fascia
❑ 97. Has a vestigial ligamentous attachment
❑ 98. Has a compound articulation with a secondary cartilaginous joint
❑ 99. Crosses the midline
❑ 100. Has the carina located in the plane
❑ 101. Meet in the midline
❑ 102. Receives the azygos vein

Theme: Blood

A   Fresh frozen plasma
B   Streptokinase
C   Aspirin
D   Heparin
E   Warfarin
F   Aprotinin
G   Vitamin K

For each set of observations below, select the most appropriate drug or product from the list of options above. Each option may be used once, more than once or not at all.

☐   103. Inhibits platelet aggregation
☐   104. Prolongs prothrombin time
☐   105. Is an inhibitor of fibrinolysis
☐   106. Is a major source of clotting factors
☐   107. Fractionated forms are more efficacious

Theme: Interpretation of the laboratory features of inherited coagulation disorders

A   Haemophilia A
B   von Willebrand's disease
C   Factor VII deficiency
D   Factor X deficiency
E   Glanzmann's disease

For each set of results below, select the most likely cause for the clotting abnormalities from the list above. Each option may be used once, more than once or not at all.

Normal ranges:
Prothrombin time (PT)   12-16 s
Activated partial thromboplastin time (APTT)   26-38 s
Platelet count (Plts)   150-400 x10⁹/l

☐   108. PT 12 s, APTT 56 s, Plts 70
☐   109. PT 45 s, APTT 28 s, Plts 345
☐   110. PT 16 s, APTT 62 s, Plts 380
☐   111. PT 35 s, APTT 45 s, Plts 321

QUESTIONS – Core Paper 1

18

Theme: Renal failure

A   Oliguria
B   Hypercalcaemia
C   Acute tubular necrosis
D   Cortical necrosis
E   Hyperkalaemia
F   Pre-renal renal failure
G   Hypertension
H   Pulmonary oedema
I   Pelviureteric junction obstruction

For each of the statements below select the most appropriate diagnosis from the list above. Each option may be used once, more than once or not at all.

❑   112. A 29-year-old man is trapped in a car involved in an RTA and sustains a prolonged period of hypotension. He is oliguric on admission and becomes anuric over the next few hours. He requires dialysis for six days and over the next four days his renal function gradually returns to normal.

❑   113. An 80-year-old with a bowel perforation required three litres of crystalloid to correct his blood pressure and improve perfusion. As his haemoglobin was 8 g/dl pre-operatively, he was transfused with three units of packed cells over four hours. During the final unit, he becomes hypoxic and confused.

❑   114. A 35-year-old woman is admitted with a lacerated liver and perforated duodenum. Her urine output was initially 12 ml/hour but following two litres of saline and two units of blood, it increases to 110 ml/hour.

Theme: Cerebral Injury

A Subdural haematoma
B Subarachnoid haemorrhage
C Diffuse axonal injury
D Extradural haematoma
E Basal skull fracture
F Intraventricular haemorrhage

For each of the patients below, select the form of cerebral injury from the list above which most closely matches the clinical scenario. Each option may be used once, more than once or not at all.

❑ 115. A 28-year-old female unrestrained, front seat car passenger hits the windscreen. She has an obvious broken nose and teeth. Bleeding from the nose, mouth and right ear is noted. She is conscious and has a GCS of 14.

❑ 116. A 40-year-old obese man with sudden onset of severe occipital headache.

❑ 117. An elderly man attends A&E having fallen a week before. He now has a fluctuating level of consciousness.

❑ 118. A 14-year-old female falls off her bicycle. She had initial loss of consciousness for ten mins, then apparently normal for one hour, followed by a deteriorating level of consciousness.

Theme: Ventilation

A PEEP
B CPAP
C Intermittent mandatory ventilation
D High frequency jet insufflation
E Pressure controlled ventilation
F Volume controlled ventilation
G Minute volume divided ventilation
H Reversed I:E ratio

For each of the statements below, select the most appropriate mode of ventilation from the list above. Each option may be used once, more than once or not at all.

☐ 119. Application of positive airway pressure throughout all phases of spontaneous ventilation.

☐ 120. Can be used to improve oxygenation in respiratory failure in addition to PEEP.

☐ 121. Tidal volume of up to 150 ml, cycled at 60–600/min, ventilation often delivered via a cannula inserted through the cricothyroid membrane.

☐ 122. Ventilator mode best used to provide a fixed tidal volume.

☐ 123. Ventilation best used to expand poorly compliant lungs.

☐ 124. May be used to reduce FiO_2 requirement and improve oxygenation.

☐ 125. A pre-set minute volume is delivered by the ventilator, but the patient is allowed to breathe spontaneously between ventilator breaths.

Theme: Cardiovascular physiology

A   End of phase 2
B   Start of phase 2
C   Throughout phase 5
D   Phase 1
E   Phase 3
F   During phases 1 and 2
G   Phase 4

For each of the events listed below, select the correct part of the cardiac cycle from the list above. Each option may be used once, more than once or not at all.

☐   126. Passive left ventricular filling
☐   127. Closure of the mitral valve
☐   128. Opening of the aortic valve
☐   129. Second heart sound
☐   130. Left ventricular ejection
☐   131. The QRS complex

END OF CORE PAPER 1

CORE PAPER 2
SECTION 1 – MCQS

1.   Atrial natriuretic peptide

❏   A   increases urine flow through vasoconstriction of the efferent arteriole
❏   B   raises GFR
❏   C   reduces water intake
❏   D   lowers renin production
❏   E   is effective in the treatment of acute tubular necrosis

2.   Regarding haemorrhage

❏   A   this is defined as acute or chronic loss of circulating blood
❏   B   the normal adult blood volume is approximately 7% of body weight
❏   C   the blood volume of obese patients is estimated on their ideal body weight
❏   D   the blood volume of children is approximately 15% of body weight
❏   E   tachycardia is the earliest measurable sign

3.   Criteria required for diagnosis of ARDS include

❏   A   changes on chest X-ray
❏   B   wedge pressure above 18 mmHg
❏   C FiO_2 of 1.0
❏   D   multiple organ failure
❏   E $pO_2 < 5$ kPa

23

4. **Clinical indicators suggestive of acute inhalational injury include**

    ❏ A   dysphagia
    ❏ B   carbonaceous sputum
    ❏ C   oesophageal carbon deposits
    ❏ D   singeing of eyebrows
    ❏ E   subcutaneous emphysema

5. **Essential components of total parenteral nutrition include**

    ❏ A   emulsifiers
    ❏ B   nitrogen
    ❏ C   fibrinogen
    ❏ D   carbohydrate
    ❏ E   acetic acid

6. **The following may reduce intra-operative heat loss**

    ❏ A   condenser-humidifier in the breathing circuit
    ❏ B   low-flow anaesthesia
    ❏ C   laminar flow in an orthopaedic theatre
    ❏ D   use of a 'bowel bag' during laparotomy
    ❏ E   use of volatile surgical preparation sterilising agents

7. **In diabetic emergencies**

    ❏ A   hypoglycaemia most commonly occurs in Type II diabetes
    ❏ B   diabetic ketoacidosis is a typical feature of Type II diabetes
    ❏ C   hyperosmolar coma is usually caused by ketoacidosis
    ❏ D   if the cause of coma is not known, insulin should be given
           until the diagnosis is confirmed
    ❏ E   glucose is useful in the initial treatment of diabetic
           ketoacidosis

8. **In shock states where SVR represents systemic vascular resistance, CO represents cardiac output and CI is cardiac index**

❑   A   septic shock produces a high SVR and high CO
❑   B   cardiogenic shock produces a low SVR and low CO
❑   C   neurogenic shock produces a low SVR and high CO
❑   D   anaphylactic shock produces a very low lactic acid level
❑   E   septic shock produces a low SVR and high CO

9. **Which of the following are true of post-operative complications:**

❑   A   the commonest cause of hyponatraemia is increased renal sodium loss
❑   B   hypoxia may occur only in the first 24 hrs after surgery
❑   C   cold, clammy peripheries may be seen in septic shock
❑   D   pneumonia should be suspected if tachypnoea, pyrexia and tachycardia appear in the first 24 hrs
❑   E   myocardial infarction is more common in post-operative patients with uncontrolled hypertension

10. **Human albumin solution**

❑   A   may induce hypernatraemia
❑   B   is most commonly used for acute volume replacement
❑   C   is stored at room temperature
❑   D   is manufactured as a bacterial recombinant protein
❑   E   may be useful in the treatment of ascites in chronic liver disease

11. **Contraindications to curative surgery in patients with non-small cell lung cancer include**

❑   A   malignant pleural effusion
❑   B   superior vena cava syndrome
❑   C   contralateral lung metastasis
❑   D   tumour < 3 cm in diameter
❑   E $FEV_1 < 3$ l

25

12. **Infectious causes of abdominal pain in HIV-infected individuals include**

❏ A cryptosporidium
❏ B cytomegalovirus
❏ C *Clostridium perfringens*
❏ D Kaposi's sarcoma
❏ E *Mycobacterium tuberculosis*

13. **Regarding hydatid disease**

❏ A the causative bacteria is *Echinococcus granulosus*
❏ B humans are accidental intermediate hosts
❏ C the normal intermediate host is the dog
❏ D hepatic lesions are often asymptomatic
❏ E diagnosis is made on needle aspiration of suspected lesions

14. **With regard to Osteomyelitis**

❏ A most commonly arises in adults from a haematogenous infection from a primary focus elsewhere in the body
❏ B *E. coli* is the commonest organism in neonates and children
❏ C in adults is most commonly due to staphylococcus
❏ D X-rays of affected bones may be normal for up to 14 days after the onset of symptoms
❏ E early high dose intravenous antibiotics are part of the treatment regimen

15. **Clostridium difficile infection**

❏ A may be adequately treated with a single dose of oral metronidazole
❏ B is usually diagnosed by Gram staining of the faeces
❏ C may be adequately treated with iv vancomycin
❏ D should be followed-up by stool culture from asymptomatic patients
❏ E may lead to colonic perforation

16. **Sterilisation of surgical equipment**

❑ A chemical sterilisation is appropriate for equipment not suitable for exposure to steam
❑ B 2% glutaraldehyde can be used for plastic equipment
❑ C dry heat sterilisation may be appropriate for equipment that is not well penetrated by steam
❑ D steam heat autoclaving is effective for rapid sterilisation of instruments

17. **When performing an incisional biopsy of a suspected large cutaneous squamous cell carcinoma**

❑ A tissue should be taken from the junction of abnormal and normal tissue
❑ B tissue from the centre of the lesion is the most likely to yield a histological diagnosis
❑ C multiple biopsies may be required to make a diagnosis
❑ D a single benign biopsy excludes a malignant lesion

18. **The primary survey of a seriously injured trauma patient includes**

❑ A airway maintenance with cervical spine control
❑ B brief neurological examination
❑ C abdominal assessment
❑ D musculoskeletal assessment
❑ E an assessment of pelvic stability

19. **The secondary survey of a severely injured patient**

❑ A only begins after the primary survey has been completed and resuscitation of life-threatening conditions has begun
❑ B includes scoring on the Glasgow Coma Scale (GCS)
❑ C includes chest, cervical spine and pelvic X-rays
❑ D does not include diagnostic peritoneal lavage
❑ E includes rectal examination

20. **In pelvic trauma**

- ❏ A pelvic fractures are usually isolated injuries
- ❏ B haemorrhage is usually arterial in nature
- ❏ C mortality of open pelvic fractures approaches 50%
- ❏ D a single view cystogram will exclude a bladder rupture
- ❏ E pelvic vascular embolization is the preferred operative approach for haemostasis
- ❏ F penile meatal blood is an indication for retrograde urethrography

21. **Acute traumatic diaphragmatic rupture**

- ❏ A is more frequent on the right side
- ❏ B is often associated with mediastinal displacement
- ❏ C may cause strangulation of abdominal viscera
- ❏ D is usually treated surgically

22. **Regarding gunshot wounds to the abdomen**

- ❏ A they should be managed non-operatively
- ❏ B high velocity bullets can result in tissue necrosis distant from the bullet track
- ❏ C they show significant visceral injury in 40% of cases
- ❏ D if an exit wound is absent, AXRs may help determine missile trajectory
- ❏ E broad spectrum antibiotics should be avoided to prevent organism resistance

23. **Burns cause tissue damage by**

- ❏ A reducing cellular metabolism
- ❏ B activating thermo-labile enzymes
- ❏ C producing vascular injury
- ❏ D denaturing protein
- ❏ E causing hyaline membrane formation

24. **Regarding skin grafts**

- ❑ A full thickness grafts contain epidermis, papillary and reticular dermis
- ❑ B full thickness grafts have lower metabolic demands compared with split skin grafts
- ❑ C split skin grafts are superior to full thickness grafts as they do not cause wound contraction
- ❑ D split skin grafts heal by re-epithelialisation
- ❑ E post-auricular skin is a useful donor site for split skin grafts

25. **A femoral nerve injury would result in**

- ❑ A absence of the knee jerk reflex
- ❑ B anaesthesia over the anterior skin of the calf
- ❑ C absence of the cremasteric reflex
- ❑ D paraesthesia of the skin over the medial malleolus
- ❑ E paraesthesia over the entire L2 dermatome

26. **The management of severe anaphylactic shock may include**

- ❑ A airway maintenance and oxygen
- ❑ B iv fluids
- ❑ C intra-arterial adrenaline
- ❑ D nebulised bronchoconstrictors
- ❑ E β-blockers

27. **Familial Adenomatous Polyposis (FAP)**

- ❑ A is inherited as an autosomal recessive disease
- ❑ B is associated with chromosomal abnormalities on chromosome 5
- ❑ C has an incidence of about 1:500 live births
- ❑ D arises as new mutations without a positive family history in approximately 30% of cases
- ❑ E has a lifetime risk of 100% of developing colorectal cancer

28. With regards to surgery for breast cancer, which of the following are relative indications for mastectomy rather than conservative breast excision:

❑ A   larger breasts
❑ B   extensive ductal carcinoma in situ (DCIS)
❑ C   impalpable disease
❑ D   salvage surgery
❑ E   axillary lymph node involvement

29. Concerning malignant melanoma

❑ A   elective regional lymph node dissection has been clearly shown to increase survival
❑ B   en bloc excision of involved regional lymph nodes is recommended in the absence of distant spread
❑ C   it responds well to chemotherapy
❑ D   it has a 60–70% 5-year survival when associated with excision of solitary metastases
❑ E   it is highly radiosensitive

30. Colorectal cancer screening for low risk groups

❑ A   testing for faecal occult blood has never been shown to increase the detection of colorectal tumours confined to the bowel wall
❑ B   compliance rates of reported faecal occult blood testing (FOBT) screening studies is of the order of 30–50%
❑ C   the optimal period between repeat testing has yet to be established
❑ D   patients should be on a high roughage, meat-free diet for 24 hours prior to testing
❑ E   the haemoccult FOBT relies on a transaminase reaction to produce a positive result

31.   **Paget's disease of the nipple**

❏   A   usually presents as a unilateral nipple nodule
❏   B   is associated with an underlying ductal breast carcinoma in
         about 50% of cases
❏   C   associated breast carcinomas have a better overall prognosis
         than breast cancer in the general population
❏   D   has a 30% incidence of coincident contralateral breast cancer
         at the time of diagnosis
❏   E   is diagnosed on clinical grounds alone

32.   **Injury to the radial nerve in the radial (spiral) groove of the
         humerus causes loss of**

❏   A   abduction of the thumb
❏   B   extension of the forearm
❏   C   supination
❏   D   cutaneous sensation over the dorsal surface of the first web
         space
❏   E   the brachioradialis tendon reflex

33.   **After damage to the ulnar nerve at the elbow, there is**

❏   A   anaesthesia over the skin of the thenar eminence
❏   B   loss of abduction of the index finger
❏   C   loss of adduction of the wrist
❏   D   loss of flexion of the little finger
❏   E   claw hand

34.   **Branches of the subclavian arteries supply the**

❏   A   thyroid gland
❏   B   breast
❏   C   rectus abdominis muscle
❏   D   brain stem
❏   E   diaphragm

35. **The sympathetic chain**

❏ A   lies on the heads of the ribs
❏ B   lies anterior to the posterior intercostal vessels
❏ C   lies medial to the splanchnic nerves
❏ D   receives white rami communicantes from all thoracic nerve roots
❏ E   passes into the abdomen behind the lateral arcuate ligament

36. **The right coronary artery**

❏ A   originates in the anterior aortic sinus
❏ B   is overlain by the right atrial appendage
❏ C   supplies the sinoatrial node
❏ D   lies on the infundibulum of the right ventricle
❏ E   anastomoses with branches of the left coronary artery

37. **The trachea**

❏ A   is palpable
❏ B   bifurcates behind the manubriosternal joint
❏ C   has a left main bronchus more vertical than the right
❏ D   has a left main bronchus which branches outside the hilum
❏ E   is innervated by the recurrent laryngeal nerve

38. **The haematological consequences of splenectomy include**

❏ A   a thrombocytosis peaking between 3–4 months
❏ B   increased circulating Howell-Jolly bodies
❏ C   reduction in circulating sideroblasts
❏ D   a leucocytosis within hours after operation
❏ E   reduced platelet adhesiveness

39. The following conditions may be associated with a microcytic anaemia:

- ❏ A β-thalassaemia
- ❏ B carcinoma of the rectum
- ❏ C hereditary haemochromatosis
- ❏ D menorrhagia
- ❏ E chronic renal failure

40. Anaemia with a normal mean cell volume may indicate

- ❏ A a combined iron and B_{12} deficiency
- ❏ B acute renal failure
- ❏ C rheumatoid arthritis
- ❏ D coeliac disease
- ❏ E folate deficiency

41. In the investigation of bleeding disorders

- ❏ A bleeding time may be prolonged in patients receiving aspirin
- ❏ B fibrinogen concentration is increased in sepsis
- ❏ C bleeding time correlates well with the severity of surgical bleeding
- ❏ D fibrinogen levels increase in disseminated intravascular coagulation
- ❏ E thrombin time is reduced in heparin therapy

42. von Willebrand's disease

- ❏ A is a sex-linked disorder
- ❏ B is the commonest inherited bleeding disorder in surgical practice
- ❏ C is associated with haemarthroses
- ❏ D manifests as a prolonged APTT and bleeding time
- ❏ E affected individuals may benefit from pre-operative desmopressin

43. Platelets for transfusion

- ☐ A are pooled from 4–6 individual donations
- ☐ B have a shelf life of four weeks after donation
- ☐ C may cause an immune mediated transfusion reaction
- ☐ D must be ABO and rhesus D crossmatched

44. Possible complications of blood transfusion include

- ☐ A graft versus host disease
- ☐ B an increased risk of recurrent malignancy
- ☐ C pancreatic endocrine insufficiency
- ☐ D life-threatening thrombocytopenia
- ☐ E T-cell leukaemia

45. The following are donation criteria for autologous transfusion:

- ☐ A a haemoglobin of greater than 11 g/dl
- ☐ B infection
- ☐ C procedures where blood loss is expected
- ☐ D ischaemic heart disease
- ☐ E immunosuppression

46. In statistical analysis

- ☐ A the mean of a set of values is the same as the standard error
- ☐ B the median of a set of values is the same as the average
- ☐ C standard deviation is a measure of the variability of a set of values
- ☐ D parametric tests are used for the assessment of data that follows a non-Gaussian distribution
- ☐ E the outcome of a rank or score (e.g. Ranson's score) cannot be Gaussian in distribution

Theme: Suture material

A   Absorbable, braided, synthetic
B   Absorbable, monofilament, synthetic
C   Nonabsorbable, braided, natural material
D   Nonabsorbable, monofilament, synthetic

For each of the suture materials listed below, select the most appropriate description from the list above. Each option may be used once, more than once, or not at all.

☐ 61. Polyglactic acid (Vicryl)
☐ 62. Nylon
☐ 63. Polyglyconate (Maxon)
☐ 64. Polypropylene (Prolene)
☐ 65. Polydioxanone (PDS)
☐ 66. Polyglycolic acid (Dexon)
☐ 67. Silk

Theme: Chemotherapy agents

A   Anti-metabolites
B   Alkylating agents
C   Corticosteroids
D   Anti-cytotoxic

For each of the drugs listed below, select the correct group of immunosuppressive agents they belong to from the list above. Each option may be used once, more than once, or not at all.

☐ 68. Cyclophosphamide
☐ 69. Methylprednisolone
☐ 70. Azathioprine
☐ 71. Cyclosporin
☐ 72. 6-mercaptopurine

Theme: Cancer therapy options

A   Radiotherapy, with steroids
B   Hormonal manipulation
C   Systemic chemotherapy
D   Surgical resection

For each of the clinical scenarios listed below, select the most appropriate management options from the list above. Each option may be used once, more than once, or not at all.

☐   73.   Recurrent non-Hodgkin's lymphoma
☐   74.   Isolated pulmonary metastasis from colorectal cancer
☐   75.   Residual anal squamous cell carcinoma (SCC) after local radiotherapy
☐   76.   Metastatic prostatic carcinoma not involving bone
☐   77.   Diffuse intracranial metastatic melanoma

Theme: Mediastinal masses

A   Superior mediastinum
B   Anterior mediastinum
C   Middle mediastinum
D   Posterior mediastinum

For each of the pathologies listed below, select the correct part of the mediastinum in which they are found from the list above. Each option may be used once, more than once, or not at all.

☐   78.   Thymic lesions
☐   79.   Neural tumours
☐   80.   Thyroid mass
☐   81.   Lymphoma
☐   82.   Bronchogenic cyst

Theme: Malignant melanoma

A   Superficial spreading melanoma
B   Acral lentiginous melanoma
C   Lentigo maligna melanoma
D   Nodular melanoma
E   Amelanotic melanoma

For each of the scenarios given below, select the correct type of cutaneous malignant melanoma from the list above. Each option may be used once, more than once, or not at all.

❑   83.   Occurs within a Hutchinson's melanotic freckle
❑   84.   Has a predilection for sites with thick epidermis such as the sole of the foot
❑   85.   Usually occurs on the face of elderly patients
❑   86.   Is the commonest type of cutaneous malignant melanoma

Theme: Resuscitation

A   Blood pressure   70/40 mmHg
B   Blood pressure   100/65 mmHg
C   Blood pressure   125/80 mmHg
D   Pulse   68/min
E   Pulse   100/min
F   Pulse   158/min
G   Respiratory rate   8/min
H   Respiratory rate   13/min
I   Respiratory rate   18/min
J   Respiratory rate   26/min
K   Respiratory rate   60/min

Select the value from the list above which would be the most likely to be considered as normal in the healthy, resting children described below. Each option may be used once, more than once or not at all.

❑   87.   Pulse in a term neonate
❑   88.   Blood pressure in a 2-year-old
❑   89.   Pulse in a 7-year-old
❑   90.   Blood pressure in a term neonate
❑   91.   Respiratory rate in a 4-year-old
❑   92.   Respiratory rate in a 12-year-old

Theme: Anatomy of the cerebral vasculature

A Posterior cerebral artery
B Posterior inferior cerebellar artery
C Internal carotid artery
D Middle meningeal artery
E Vertebral artery
F Basilar artery
G Striate arteries
H Middle cerebral artery

For each patient with neurological abnormalities below, select the artery most likely to be affected from the list above. Each option may be used once, more than once or not at all.

☐ 93. A 75-year-old man wakes one morning with a hemiparesis, and loss of discriminatory touch, movement and vibration, all on the left side. On protrusion, his tongue deviates to the right.

☐ 94. A 76-year-old man wakes one morning with absence of pain and temperature sensation over the right side of the body, dysarthria and dysphagia. There is also loss of pain and temperature sensation over the area of distribution of the left trigeminal nerve.

☐ 95. A 74-year-old man notices that he collides with objects on his right side, but he is able to read. His perimetry charts show that he has a complete right homonymous hemianopia with macular sparing.

☐ 96. A 76-year-old man suddenly collapses. When he recovers consciousness, he is found to have a complete right hemiparesis, complete right-sided anaesthesia, aphasia, and paralysis of his right lower facial musculature. There is also a right homonymous hemianopia.

Theme: Anatomy of the heart

A   Right coronary artery
B   Coronary sinus
C   Membranous interventricular septum
D   Moderator band
E   Septal cusp of the tricuspid valve
F   Anterior cusp of the mitral valve
G   Muscular interventricular septum
H   Interatrial septum
I   Sulcus terminalis
J   Left atrial appendage
K   Oblique pericardial sinus
L   Infundibulum

For each of the statements below, select the most likely option from the list above. Each option may be used once, more than once or not at all.

❏   97. Location of the sinoatrial node
❏   98. Originates from the anterior aortic sinus
❏   99. Overlies the left coronary artery
❏   100. Drains into the right atrium
❏   101. Is connected to the largest papillary muscle
❏   102. Lies posterior to the left atrium
❏   103. Location of the bundle of His
❏   104. Location of the atrioventricular node

Theme: Interpretation of the full blood count

A   Myelofibrosis
B   Chronic lymphocytic leukaemia
C   Idiopathic thrombocytopenic purpura (ITP)
D   Leukaemoid reaction
E   Polycythaemia rubra vera

For each set of results below, select the most likely diagnosis from the list of options above. Each option may be used once, more than once or not at all.

Normal ranges:

Haemoglobin (Hb)	12–17 g/dl
White cell count (WBC)	4–11 x10^9/l
Neutrophils (N)	3.5–7.5 x 10^9/l
Lymphocytes (L)	1.5–4.5 x 10^9/l
Platelets (Plt)	150–400 x10^9/l

- [ ] 105. Hb 21.3   WBC 14 (N 10, L 4)   Plt 490
- [ ] 106. Hb 12.2   WBC 298 (N 2, L 296)   Plt 160
- [ ] 107. Hb 14.5   WBC 5.4 (N 3.8, L 1.3)   Plt 25
- [ ] 108. Hb 9.8   WBC 1.1 (N 0.5, L 0.6)   Plt 45
- [ ] 109. Hb 13.5   WBC 98 (N 82, L 16)   Plt 640

Theme: Anticoagulant treatment regimens

A   Warfarin to maintain an INR of 2.0–3.0
B   Unfractionated heparin 5000 iu subcutaneously *bd.*
C   Unfractionated heparin intravenously to maintain an APTT ratio of 2.5–3.5
D   Tinzaparin 3500 u/kg *od.*
E   Tinzaparin 175 u/kg *od.*

For each of the clinical scenarios listed below, select the most appropriate anticoagulation regime to initiate treatment from the list of options above. Each option may be used once, more than once or not at all.

❏   110. A 34-year-old woman with factor V Leiden but no previous history of venous thrombosis is admitted for correction of hallux valgus. A previous hallux valgus procedure was complicated by excessive bleeding.

❏   111. A 67-year-old woman develops a popliteal vein thrombosis five days after a total hip replacement.

❏   112. A 45-year-old man takes warfarin for a prosthetic mitral valve and attends the ward three days before an elective pancreatectomy.

Theme: Electrolyte disturbances

A   Mannitol
B   Fluid restriction
C   Blood
D   Dopamine
E   5% dextrose
F   8.4% sodium bicarbonate
G   Haemofiltration
H   0.9% saline

For each of the patients below, select the most appropriate treatment from the list above. Each option may be used once, more than once or not at all.

❏ 113. A 60-year-old post-operative aortic aneurysm repair, ventilated because of pneumonia. His electrolyte picture is Na$^+$ 123 mmol/l, K$^+$ 4.7 mmol/l, Urea 3.4 mmol/l, Creatinine 96 μmol/l, HCO$_3^-$ 24 mmol/l.

❏ 114. A 24-year-old post-operative perforated appendix with peritonitis develops septicaemia. Despite adequate restoration of her circulating volume, she becomes anuric and fails to respond to 120 mg frusemide. Her electrolyte picture is Na$^+$ 128 mmol/l, K$^+$ 7.4 mmol/l, Urea 28.6 mmol/l, Creatinine 940 μmol/l, HCO$_3^-$ 16.4 mmol/l.

❏ 115. A 7-year-old boy with head injury with cerebral oedema due to diffuse axonal injury develops polyuria. His electrolyte picture is Na$^+$ 150 mmol/l, K$^+$ 5.8 mmol/l, Urea 14.4 mmol/l, Creatinine 90 μmol/l, HCO$_3^-$ 20 mmol/l.

Theme: Respiratory Physiology

A Compliance
B Functional Residual Capacity
C PEEP
D Vital capacity
E Tidal volume
F FEV_1
G Dead space
H Shunt
I West's zones
J Starling resistor
K Minute volume

For each of the definitions below, select the most appropriate term from the list above. Each option may be used once, more than once or not at all.

❑ 116. Volume change per unit pressure change – a measure of distensibility
❑ 117. Theoretical regions of lung tissue which demonstrate different effects of gravity on the regional alveoli and corresponding pulmonary circulation
❑ 118. The sum of residual volume and expiratory reserve volume
❑ 119. The volume forcibly exhaled from full inspiration in one second
❑ 120. An amount of venous blood which bypasses ventilated alveoli
❑ 121. Volume of inspired air which takes no part in gas exchange
❑ 122. Model of a length of collapsible tubing in a rigid box which is used to demonstrate the effects of gravity on regional pulmonary circulation
❑ 123. The largest volume that can be expired after a maximal inspiration

Theme: Monitoring in neurosurgical ITU

A   Intracranial pressure (IPP)
B   Cerebral perfusion pressure (CPP)
C   Mean arterial blood pressure (MAP)
D   Central venous pressure (CVP)
E   Transcranial Doppler sonography
F   Near-infrared spectroscopy
G   Glasgow Coma Scale (GCS)

For each of the statements below, select the most appropriate monitoring modality from the list above. Each option may be used once, more than once or not at all.

❏   124. Is equal to the sum of the CPP and ICP
❏   125. Measures flow velocity in vessels
❏   126. Allows global estimation of cerebral blood volume and oxygenation
❏   127. Can be calculated from the MAP and ICP

Theme: Spinal trauma

A   Right posterior column
B   Spinothalamic tract
C   Corticospinal tract
D   Cerebral
E   Left posterior column
F   Medulla
G   Cauda equina
H   Cervical cord injury

For each of the clinical presentations below, select the most likely neurological injury from the list above. Each option may be used once, more than once or not at all.

❏   128. A young man is admitted after a high velocity traffic accident. He is unconscious with flaccid areflexia and flaccid anal sphincter. He has diaphragmatic breathing and priapism.
❏   129. A woman is admitted after having been hit by a car when crossing a busy road. She is complaining of pain between her shoulders. She is found to have lost position sense of her left toes and vibration sensation of her left foot.

END OF CORE PAPER 2

Time allowed: 2 hours
Indicate your answers in the spaces provided

CORE PAPER 3
SECTION 1 – MCQS

1.   **The catabolic phase of the metabolic response to injury**

❑   A   is accompanied by increased energy expenditure
❑   B   is accompanied by a positive nitrogen balance
❑   C   varies in response to the severity of the trauma
❑   D   is most dramatic following multi-system trauma and extensive burns
❑   E   is prolonged by sepsis

2.   **Consequences of major burns include**

❑   A   reduced RBC survival
❑   B   disseminated intravascular coagulation
❑   C   myocardial suppression
❑   D   late thrombocytosis
❑   E   eosinophilia

3.   **A rapid loss of 25% of the blood volume will**

❑   A   increase ADH levels
❑   B   activate the renin-angiotensin system
❑   C   stimulate thirst
❑   D   produce a fall in blood glucose
❑   E   produce hyperkalaemia

4.   **Renal blood flow**

❑   A   may be reduced by 50% in acute renal failure
❑   B   is normally kept constant by autoregulation
❑   C   is higher in the medulla than in the cortex
❑   D   is unaffected by hypertension

5.   **A tracheostomy will reduce**

❑ A   vital capacity
❑ B   functional residual capacity
❑ C   physiological dead space
❑ D   airway resistance
❑ E   dynamic lung compliance

6.   **Drugs known to cause renal failure include the following:**

❑ A   mannitol
❑ B   β-blockers
❑ C   thyroxine
❑ D   ciprofloxacin
❑ E   vancomycin

7.   **The following are indicators of regional blood flow:**

❑ A   cardiac output measurement by Swan-Ganz catheterisation
❑ B   gastric tonometry
❑ C   blood lactate
❑ D   jugular bulb oxygen saturation
❑ E   mixed venous oxygen saturation

8.   **Local host factors predisposing to wound infection include the**

❑ A   prior irradiation in the field of the wound
❑ B   length of the incision
❑ C   amount of muscle and fascia divided
❑ D   direction of the incision in relation to Langer's lines
❑ E   size of the bacterial inoculum

9. **Regarding suture materials**

- [ ] A prolene should be avoided in the urinary tract
- [ ] B catgut should be avoided in the biliary tree
- [ ] C chromic catgut has an intracorporeal half-life of two days
- [ ] D monofilament sutures give superior functional results over braided sutures for small bowel anastomoses
- [ ] E it is best to use the smallest calibre material strong enough to hold the tissues in question

10. **Regarding skin grafts**

- [ ] A split skin grafts contain epidermis only
- [ ] B split skin grafts maintain their own blood supply
- [ ] C thinner split skin grafts are more likely to 'take' than thicker ones
- [ ] D split skin grafts result in greater contraction than full thickness grafts
- [ ] E minor degrees of recipient site bacterial contamination may inhibit a graft to 'take'

11. **Full thickness burns**

- [ ] A usually have a pale, white or leathery appearance
- [ ] B often have a weeping surface
- [ ] C are painful and sensitive
- [ ] D often have broken skin and exposed fat
- [ ] E can be caused by prolonged exposure to hot fluids

12. **Adult respiratory distress syndrome (ARDS)**

- [ ] A is occasionally due to pulmonary oedema of cardiac origin
- [ ] B promotes superoxide induced parenchymal damage
- [ ] C does not affect pulmonary ventilation/perfusion matching
- [ ] D is associated with discrete pulmonary nodules on X-ray

47

13. **Traumatic chest injuries**

❑ A usually require operation
❑ B are associated with cardiac or major vascular injury in 10% of cases
❑ C are responsible for 25% of trauma deaths
❑ D producing sternal fractures may be associated with cardiac arrhythmias
❑ E producing tracheal rupture are usually amenable to surgical repair with good outcome

14. **Penetrating lower chest wounds**

❑ A may be associated with false aneurysm formation
❑ B are associated with a significant intra-abdominal organ injury in 5% of lower chest stab wounds
❑ C are associated with a significant intra-abdominal organ injury in 60% of lower chest gunshot wounds
❑ D can usually be managed without the use of chest drainage

15. **In the critically injured patient**

❑ A a tension pneumothorax should be confirmed radiologically prior to thoracocentesis
❑ B airway patency ensures adequate ventilation
❑ C a flail chest is a frequently missed diagnosis that compromises ventilation
❑ D tracheal intubation is indicated for the unconscious patient
❑ E cardiac tamponade will reliably give rise to distended neck veins

16. **Clinical signs of significant injury in penetrating neck trauma include**

❑ A expanding haematoma
❑ B dysphonia
❑ C exophthalmos
❑ D dysphagia
❑ E haemoptysis

17.   Accepted diagnostic peritoneal lavage criteria indicating need
        for laparotomy include

❏   A   catheter drainage of bile
❏   B   catheter aspiration of 5 ml of clear fluid
❏   C   lavage fluid exiting via a chest drain
❏   D   laboratory analysis of peritoneal lavage fluid (unspun) of
        > 500 RBCs/mm³
❏   E   laboratory analysis of peritoneal lavage fluid (unspun) of
        > 500 WBCs/mm³

18.   Traction injury of the upper trunk of the brachial plexus
        results in

❏   A   loss of medial rotation of the arm
❏   B   paralysis of the deltoid muscle
❏   C   loss of cutaneous sensation over the lateral surface of the arm
❏   D   loss of supination
❏   E   extension of the forearm

19.   After damage to the common peroneal nerve there is

❏   A   failure of the foot to clear the ground on walking
❏   B   loss of cutaneous sensation over the sole of the foot
❏   C   weakness of inversion of the foot
❏   D   wasting of muscles in the anterior compartment of the calf
❏   E   collapse of the transverse arch of the foot

20.   Chronic subdural haematoma

❏   A   is usually produced by injury to the middle meningeal artery
❏   B   is rarely bilateral
❏   C   may not be present for several months
❏   D   usually produces papilloedema
❏   E   may occur after apparent trivial injury

21. In faecal occult blood test (FOBT) screening with Haemoccult

- A false negatives may result from ingestion of animal haemoglobin
- B false positives may result from ingestion of certain vegetables due to their folic acid content
- C screen detected tumours are more likely to be at an earlier stage than symptomatic disease
- D it has been shown to give a 15–30% reduction in incidence in colorectal cancer specific mortality
- E approximately 40% of patients with a positive test will on investigation turn out to have a colorectal carcinoma

22. In the outcome of treatment for breast cancer

- A radical mastectomy has been shown to give better survival than modified radical mastectomy
- B post-operative radiotherapy following modified radical mastectomy prolongs the disease-free interval and survival
- C adjuvant chemotherapy appears to prolong the disease-free interval in pre-menopausal women with positive lymph nodes
- D tamoxifen appears to increase the disease-free interval in post-menopausal women with oestrogen-positive tumours
- E lumpectomy, radiotherapy, and nodal sampling achieve results equivalent to modified radical mastectomy

23. Lesions which may predispose to oesophageal carcinoma

- A oesophageal webs
- B pharyngeal pouches
- C corrosive oesophagitis
- D achalasia
- E oesophageal varices

24. **Gastric cancer may present with**

❑ A   Krukenberg's tumour
❑ B   Bloomer's shelf
❑ C   Curling's ulcer
❑ D   a positive Courvoisier's sign
❑ E   Virchow's node

25. **Carcinoid tumours**

❑ A   of the small bowel often behave in a malignant fashion
❑ B   are usually slow growing
❑ C   prognosis is independent of the size of the primary
❑ D   produce the carcinoid syndrome by releasing catecholamines
❑ E   are associated with increased urinary 5-HIAA excretion

26. **Risk factors for the development of breast cancer include**

❑ A   previous fibroadenoma
❑ B   nulliparity
❑ C   contralateral breast cancer
❑ D   increasing age
❑ E   mammary duct ectasia

27. **In blunt head trauma**

❑ A   the duration of post-traumatic amnesia correlates well with the degree of primary brain injury
❑ B   the duration of retrograde amnesia correlates well with the degree of primary brain injury
❑ C   depressed conscious level in a patient with a blood alcohol level over 300 mg/dl can safely be attributed to alcohol intoxication
❑ D   codeine phosphate analgesia must be avoided
❑ E   in a comatose patient with multiple injuries, haemodynamic stabilisation takes priority over evacuation of intracranial haematoma

28. In the diagnosis and treatment of compartment syndrome in the leg

☐ A absence of a fracture makes the diagnosis unlikely
☐ B compartment pressure manometry is needed to make the diagnosis
☐ C fasciotomy should be performed when the compartment pressure exceeds diastolic blood pressure
☐ D fasciotomy should be confined to the affected compartment
☐ E primary skin closure should be performed to cover the affected muscles

29. The oesophagus

☐ A is formed at the lower border of the cricoid cartilage
☐ B passes through the central tendon of the diaphragm
☐ C receives a sensory nerve supply from the phrenic nerve
☐ D lies behind the right atrium
☐ E is crossed anteriorly by the right main bronchus

30. The left phrenic nerve

☐ A carries sympathetic fibres to the diaphragm
☐ B lies on the fibrous pericardium
☐ C innervates the peritoneum
☐ D originates from the C5 segment of the spinal cord
☐ E enters the chest anterior to the subclavian vein

31. The surface of the right lung is indented by the

☐ A trachea
☐ B oesophagus
☐ C superior vena cava
☐ D right ventricle
☐ E subclavian vein

32.   **The clavipectoral fascia is**

❑ A   pierced by the basilic vein
❑ B   split to enclose the pectoralis major muscle
❑ C   pierced by the medial pectoral nerves
❑ D   overlain by the infra-clavicular lymph nodes
❑ E   overlain by the C4 dermatome

33.   **Signs of S1 nerve root compression include**

❑ A   claw toes
❑ B   weakness of extensor hallucis longus
❑ C   weakness of plantar flexion of the ankle
❑ D   weakness of ankle dorsiflexion
❑ E   enhanced ankle jerk reflex

34.   **Asplenic patients are at particulary increased risk of overwhelming sepsis from**

❑ A   anaerobic bacteria
❑ B   *Streptococcus pneumoniae*
❑ C   *Neisseria meningitidis*
❑ D   *Haemophilus influenza*
❑ E   *Bacteroides fragilis*
❑ F   fungi

35.   **Correct pairings of the organ and predominant commensal bacterial flora include**

❑ A   skin and coliforms
❑ B   lower respiratory tract and streptococci
❑ C   oropharynx and streptococci
❑ D   large bowel and *Bacteroides fragilis*
❑ E   vagina and lactobacillus

36.   Human Immunodeficiency Virus (HIV) infection

☐   A   is caused by a retrovirus
☐   B   may be diagnosed by Western blotting
☐   C   is present in high titre in the blood of asymptomatic carriers
☐   D   the risk of seroconversion following a needlestick injury from an HIV positive patient is approximately 1 in 25
☐   E   is more infectious following a needlestick injury than hepatitis B

37.   A patient presenting for elective laparoscopic cholecystectomy is taking warfarin and aspirin for atrial fibrillation and has an INR of 3

☐   A   the warfarin should be continued intra-operatively
☐   B   the aspirin should be stopped on the day before surgery
☐   C   INR is a measurement of activated partial thromboplastin time
☐   D   the patient is at an excessive risk and should not have the operation
☐   E   the patient should be given vitamin K and fresh frozen plasma to correct the INR

38.   The following conditions may be associated with a raised mean cell volume:

☐   A   dietary iron deficiency
☐   B   vegan diet
☐   C   alcoholic liver disease
☐   D   recovery from acute haemorrhage
☐   E   chronic haemolytic anaemia

39.   An AB negative patient may

☐   A   receive O negative blood
☐   B   donate blood to an O negative recipient
☐   C   receive cryoprecipitate from an AB positive donor
☐   D   have antibodies to the rhesus D antigen
☐   E   have antibodies to the Landsteiner A antigen

40. **Sickle cell disease**

- [ ] A is an example of a polygenic disorder
- [ ] B can be diagnosed by examination of the blood film
- [ ] C is associated with gallstones
- [ ] D usually causes splenomegaly
- [ ] E is associated with increased peri-operative mortality

41. **Low molecular weight heparins**

- [ ] A have a mean molecular weight of 15 kD
- [ ] B have a longer half-life than unfractionated heparins
- [ ] C act predominantly on Factor Xa
- [ ] D have a low bioavailability after subcutaneous injection
- [ ] E are predominantly eliminated by the kidney

42. **Warfarin**

- [ ] A impairs the recycling of vitamin K
- [ ] B inhibits the synthesis of fibrinogen
- [ ] C is best monitored with the APTT
- [ ] D does not affect the bioavailability of antibiotics
- [ ] E requires 24 hours to become effective

43. **The following increase the risk of peri-operative venous thrombosis:**

- [ ] A sickle cell disease
- [ ] B adenocarcinoma of the ovary
- [ ] C anti-thrombin III deficiency
- [ ] D increased age
- [ ] E ulcerative colitis

44. **Red cell donations in the United Kingdom**

☐ A may transmit cytomegalovirus
☐ B are routinely heat treated to inactivate the hepatitis B virus
☐ C may cause *Pseudomonas septicaemia*
☐ D are now guaranteed HIV-1 negative
☐ E may transmit hepatitis G

45. **Immune mediated transfusion reactions**

☐ A must be due to ABO incompatibility if haemolysis occurs
☐ B may be due to a secondary antibody response
☐ C affect more than 10–20% of red cell or platelet transfusions
☐ D may be due to plasma protein antigens
☐ E may be due to white cell antigens

46. **Plasma substitutes**

☐ A are useful in hyponatraemic hypovolaemia
☐ B contain osmotically active material with high molecular weight
☐ C do not cause anaphylactic reactions
☐ D are useful volume expanders in congestive cardiac failure
☐ E may interfere with crossmatching

47. **Which of the following statistical tests are examples of parametric tests:**

☐ A paired t-test
☐ B unpaired t-test
☐ C Wilcoxon test
☐ D Mann-Whitney test
☐ E ANOVA test

SECTION 2 – EMQs

Theme: Skin lesions

A Central keratin plug
B Keratin pearl formation
C Intra-epidermal (*in situ*) squamous carcinoma
D S-100 positive on immunohistochemical staining
E Palisading basal cells at the periphery of tumour islands

For each of the lesions listed below, select the most appropriate characteristics from the list above. Each option may be used once, more than once, or not at all.

- 61. Malignant melanoma
- 62. Basal cell carcinoma
- 63. Squamous cell carcinoma
- 64. Bowen's disease
- 65. Keratoacanthoma

Theme: Histological tumour types

A Hamartoma
B Neuroendocrine tumour
C Neoplastic polyp
D Stromal tumour

For each of the tumours/polyps listed below, select the correct histological type they belong to from the list above. Each option may be used once, more than once, or not at all.

- 66. Villous adenoma
- 67. Peutz-Jeghers polyp
- 68. Juvenile polyp
- 69. Carcinoid tumour
- 70. Insulinoma
- 71. Leiomyosarcoma
- 72. Glucagonoma

Theme: Tumour markers

A   α-fetoprotein
B   β-hCG
C   Carcinoembryonic antigen
D   Paraproteins
E   Acid phosphatase

For each of the tumours listed below, select the most appropriate serum marker from the list above. Each option may be used once, more than once, or not at all.

☐   73.   Choriocarcinoma
☐   74.   Hepatoma
☐   75.   Prostatic carcinoma
☐   76.   Colorectal cancer
☐   77.   Multiple myeloma

Theme: Pathological chest conditions

A   Pulmonary cysts
B   Bronchogenic cysts
C   Aspergilloma
D   Malignant mesothelioma
E   Idiopathic mediastinal fibrosis

For each of the clinical scenarios listed below, select the most likely lesion from the list above. Each of the options may be used once, more than once, or not at all.

☐   78.   Mycelial mass with cellular debris
☐   79.   Affects both visceral and parietal pleura
☐   80.   Connected to the airways and therefore contain air
☐   81.   Is thought to have an autoimmune aetiology
☐   82.   Usually closely related to the trachea, hilum or oesophagus

Theme: Five year survival rates of tumours

A < 5%
B 5–10%
C 25%
D 50–60%
E 80–90%
F > 95%

For each of the clinical scenarios listed below, select the most likely 5-year survival rate from the list above. Each option may be used once, more than once, or not at all.

❑ 83. Carcinoid of the vermiform appendix
❑ 84. Duke's A rectal cancer
❑ 85. Oesophageal cancer
❑ 86. Pancreatic carcinoma
❑ 87. Metastatic prostatic cancer
❑ 88. Duke's B rectal cancer
❑ 89. Carcinoid of the small bowel

53.   Theme: Cross matching of blood

A Uncrossmatched O rhesus D negative blood
B Uncrossmatched AB rhesus D negative blood
C Crossmatched A rhesus D positive blood
D Uncrossmatched AB rhesus D positive blood
E Crossmatched AB rhesus D negative blood

For each of the clinical scenarios listed below, select the most appropriate red cell product from the list above. Each option may be used once, more than once or not at all.

❑ 90. A 56-year-old man of group AB rhesus D negative, requires two units for an elective colectomy
❑ 91. A 71-year-old woman, known to be group AB rhesus D positive from a recent 'group and save' has life-threatening bleeding during a minor surgical procedure
❑ 92. A 23-year-old woman who is group AB rhesus D negative requires blood to cover an elective gynaecological procedure
❑ 93. A 19-year-old male trauma victim of unknown identity with severe intra-thoracic bleeding

Theme: Blood gas data interpretation

A   Tachypnoea, accessory muscles of respiration, intercostal recession
B   Vomiting and fluid loss from biliary fistula
C   IDDM with pneumonia
D   Cardiorespiratory arrest, during resuscitation
E   Thyrotoxicosis
F   Acetylsalicylic acid overdose
G   24 hours after major crush injury

For each of the blood results listed below, select the most likely patient from the list above. Each option may be used once, more than once or not at all.

❑ 94. pH 7.54 pO_2 12.1 kPa pCO_2 2.9 kPa Na^+ 135
          K^+ 3.1 Cl^- 128

❑ 95. pH 6.81 pO_2 73 kPa pCO_2 14.1 kPa Na^+ 142
          K+ 5.6   Cl 95

❑ 96. pH 7.49 pO_2 13.1 kPa pCO_2 4.8 kPa Na^+ 132
          K^+ 3.5 Cl^- 87

❑ 97. pH 7.16 pO_2 6.0 kPa pCO_2 12.4 kPa Na^+ 141
          K^+ 4.2 Cl^- 109

❑ 98. pH 7.26 pO_2 9.8 kPa pCO_2 4.6 kPa Na^+ 138
          K^+ 3.5 Cl^- 108

❑ 99. pH 7.29 pO_2 11.1 kPa pCO_2 3.4 kPa Na^+ 135
          K^+ 6.6 Cl^- 98

Theme: Renal Failure

A   0.9% saline
B   Labetalol infusion
C   Dopamine
D   Intravenous or nebulised salbutamol
E   Mannitol
F   5% dextrose
G   Blood
H   Rapamycin

For each of the statements below, select the most appropriate initial treatment from the list above. Each option may be used once, more than once or not at all.

☐   100. A 52-year-old with multi-system failure due to pancreatitis becomes oliguric. Laboratory analysis reveals: Na^+ 133 mmo/l, K^+ 7.4 mmol/l, Urea 22.8 mmol/l, HCO_3^- 14.7 mmol/l, Creatinine 405 μmol/l.

☐   101. A 25-year-old female with acute hydrocephalus has an external intraventricular drain inserted. There are large CSF losses.

☐   102. A 67-year-old post-operative ruptured aortic aneurysm develops oliguria and hypotension. His CVP is 20 cmH$_2$O and pulse 130/min.

Theme: Treatment of bleeding in a anti-coagulated patient

A   Cessation of anticoagulant therapy and observation
B   Intramuscular phytomenadione
C   Fresh frozen plasma 30 ml/kg alone
D   Intravenous phytomenadione and fresh frozen plasma 30 ml/kg
E   Intravenous phytomenadione alone
F   Intravenous protamine sulphate
G   Oral protamine sulphate and observation

For each of the following clinical scenarios below, select the appropriate measure to correct the haemostatic abnormality from the list above. Each option may be used once, more than once or not at all.

❑   103. A 56-year-old man who has been taking warfarin for atrial fibrillation for four years, recently received a course of oral antibiotics from his GP for a chest infection. He now presents with life-threatening rectal bleeding. His INR is 8.0.

❑   104. A 28-year-old woman with a prosthetic mitral valve has recently undergone an elective thyroidectomy. Preoperatively her warfarin was discontinued and she was established on an intravenous heparin infusion. Immediately before theatre, her INR was 1.3 and her APTT ratio was 2.0. 12 hours post-operatively she develops severe bleeding from her wound. Her INR is now 1.1 and her APTT ratio 6.0.

Theme: Trauma due to RTA

A   Frontal impact RTA
B   Side impact RTA
C   Rear impact RTA
D   Pedestrian in an RTA

For each of the traumatic injuries listed below, select the most likely scenario to produce the injuries from the list above. Each option may be used once, more than once, or not at all.

❑   105. Pelvic and acetabular fractures
❑   106. Myocardial contusion
❑   107. Lateral flail chest
❑   108. Aortic transection
❑   109. Lower limb fractures

QUESTIONS – Core Paper 3

62

Theme: Anatomy of intracranial haemorrhage/thrombosis

A   Cavernous venous sinus
B   External carotid artery
C   Middle meningeal artery
D   Sigmoid venous sinus

E   Internal carotid artery
F   Cerebral vein
G   Jugular vein
H   Cerebral artery

For each of the clinical scenarios below, select the vascular structure most likely to be involved from the list above. Each option may be used once, more than once or not at all.

❑   110.   A collapsed 30-year-old woman is admitted with acute severe epistaxis. She had been complaining for some time previously of headache and diplopia, worse on looking to the left. On examination, she has a left-sided medial strabismus and pulsation of the left eye. Fresh red blood is gushing from the nose, her pulse is racing and her BP is dropping alarmingly. No signs of raised intracranial pressure are detectable.

❑   111.   A 12-year-old girl falls from her pony, hits her head on the trunk of a fallen tree, and is knocked unconscious. She quickly recovers and feels well enough to continue the ride. That evening, she complains of headache and begins vomiting. Concerned by her increasingly detached behaviour, her father calls the doctor. She slowly drifts into unconsciousness. In A & E, she is found to be in a deep coma, with a bradycardia and mild papilloedema. Skull X-ray reveals a fracture over the left temple.

❑   112.   A 20-year-old male student comes to casualty complaining of morning headaches, which have remorselessly increased in severity and duration. Recently, his flatmate has noticed detached episodes in consciousness for which his friend has little or no recollection. Six weeks earlier the patient had bumped his head after an emergency stop whilst a passenger in his friend's car. He had hit his forehead on the windscreen, but was not knocked out and had dismissed the incident as minor. Whilst in casualty, he collapses and is unrousable. Examination reveals marked signs of raised intracranial pressure.

❑   113.   A 23-year-old man collapses whilst standing in a bus queue and is rushed to hospital without regaining consciousness. Examination confirms that he is deeply comatosed with severe signs of raised intracranial pressure, but no skull fractures.

❑   114.   A teenage girl with chronic sinusitis develops severe pain in the left eye and forehead. There is exophthalmos and oedema of the eyelids, cornea and root of the nose, associated with pyrexia, severe headache, and malaise. There is complete paralysis of all movements of the left eye.

63

Theme: Surface/radiological anatomy of the thorax

A 5th intercostal space
B Left sternoclavicular joint
C Right pulmonary artery
D Manubriosternal joint
E 4th rib
F 1st left costal cartilage
G Recurrent laryngeal nerve
H 3rd intercostal space

For each of the statements below, select the most likely landmark from the list above. Each option may be used once, more than once or not at all.

☐ 115. Inferior vena cava
☐ 116. Bifurcation of the brachiocephalic artery
☐ 117. Oblique fissure of the right lung
☐ 118. Left ventricle
☐ 119. Hilum of the lung
☐ 120. Commencement of the superior vena cava
☐ 121. Lower border of the arch of the aorta
☐ 122. Termination of the thoracic duct

Theme: Local anaesthetic agents

A Bupivacaine
B Amethocaine
C Prilocaine
D Cocaine
E Cinchocaine
F Dibucaine
G None of above

For each set of observations listed below, select the most appropriate local anaesthetic agent from the list of options above. Each option may be used once, more than once or not at all.

☐ 123. Commonly used for conjunctival anaesthesia
☐ 124. Caused several deaths when used in Bier's blocks
☐ 125. Causes sympathetic stimulation
☐ 126. Is the best agent for Bier's blocks
☐ 127. Is formulated with hyperbaric phenol

END OF CORE PAPER 3

CORE PAPER 4
SECTION 1 – MCQS

1.   **Inotropes producing peripheral vasoconstriction include**

❏ A   dopexamine
❏ B   dobutamine
❏ C   adrenaline
❏ D   isoprenaline
❏ E   noradrenaline

2.   **Changes in cellular metabolism associated with shock include**

❏ A   accumulation of lactic acid
❏ B   increased ATP production
❏ C   passage of sodium into cells
❏ D   passage of potassium into cells
❏ E   lysosomal fragmentation
❏ F   increased ketone production

3.   **Hyperbaric oxygen therapy**

❏ A   is used in the treatment of carbon monoxide poisoning
❏ B   can be applied with an anaesthetic breathing circuit
❏ C   may cause acute oxygen toxicity
❏ D   requires the use of a pressurised chamber
❏ E   typically consists of one 20 minute session

4.   **Squamous cell carcinoma**

❏ A   is associated with chemical carcinogens
❏ B   may be locally destructive
❏ C   can be treated with radiotherapy
❏ D   can be treated with topical chemotherapy
❏ E   is associated with albinism

5.   **With regard to pancreatic biopsy**

☐ A   Kocherisation of the duodenum is mandatory for trucut biopsies of the head
☐ B   it may need to be carried out by a laparotomy
☐ C   FNA cytology may allow definitive diagnosis of malignant cells
☐ D   material can be examined by frozen section
☐ E   it is associated with a 25% complication rate

6.   **Basal cell carcinomas (BCC)**

☐ A   are also known as epidermoid carcinomas
☐ B   are the commonest malignant cutaneous tumours
☐ C   are related to sunlight exposure
☐ D   may be multifocal
☐ E   undergo frequent nodal spread if >2.5 cm in diameter
☐ F   may undergo cystic change
☐ G   are locally invasive
☐ H   are usually radiosensitive

7.   **Adult Respiratory Distress Syndrome (ARDS)**

☐ A   usually requires pulmonary biopsy for diagnosis
☐ B   increases pulmonary compliance
☐ C   increases dead-space ventilation
☐ D   produces an overall mortality of approximately 90%
☐ E   prognosis is independent of other organ complications

8.   **Recognised features of cardiac tamponade include**

☐ A   a 'globular' cardiac outline on CXR
☐ B   prominent heart sounds
☐ C   collapsed neck veins
☐ D   pulsus paradoxus
☐ E   hypertension
☐ F   Charcot's triad

9.   **Diaphragmatic rupture from blunt trauma**

☐ A   occurs most commonly to the right hemi-diaphragm
☐ B   usually produces obvious initial CXR changes
☐ C   may cause abdominal visceral herniation which can be felt
         during the placement of a chest drain
☐ D   can be readily diagnosed by diagnostic peritoneal lavage
         (DPL)

10.   **Fibroadenomas of the breast**

☐ A   contain both epithelial and stromal elements
☐ B   are macroscopically encapsulated lesions
☐ C   have a significant increased risk of cancerous change
☐ D   usually regress spontaneously
☐ E   interfere with breast feeding

11.   **Gastric cancer**

☐ A   comprises adenocarcinomas in approximately 95% of cases
☐ B   is associated with a previous partial gastrectomy
☐ C   commonly causes anorexia and weight loss
☐ D   presents with a palpable abdominal mass in approximately
         50% cases

12.   **Faecal occult blood testing with Haemoccult**

☐ A   relies on a guaiac-based test detecting peroxidase-like activity
         of haematin in faeces
☐ B   reliably detects approximately 2 ml of blood passed in the
         stool per day
☐ C   has a 10% sensitivity in detecting large adenomatous polyps
☐ D   has a 20% sensitivity in detecting a colonic carcinoma
☐ E   is less likely to detect upper gastrointestinal bleeding than
         colonic bleeding

13. **With regard to viral hepatitis**

❏ A hepatitis B is not known to be vertically transmitted
❏ B hepatitis A does not produce chronic active hepatitis
❏ C the incubation period for hepatitis B is approximately
 1–6 months
❏ D the level of hepatitis B surface Antigen (sAg) in the blood rises
 before symptoms become apparent
❏ E the presence of circulating hepatitis B sAg always indicates
 active infection and infectivity

14. **Actinomycosis infection**

❏ A is most commonly found in the groin
❏ B is most commonly due to *Actinomyces propionibacterium*
❏ C usually produces positive cultures at 48 hours
❏ D produces a characteristic discharge containing sulphur
 granules
❏ E is caused by Gram-negative obligate anaerobic bacteria

15. **Concerning pulmonary tuberculosis**

❏ A it is predominantly caused by *Mycobacterium tuberculosis
 bovis*
❏ B it is usually transmitted by ingestion of infected milk
❏ C it is rising in incidence in Western countries
❏ D induced hypersensitivity reaction is mediated by B-
 lymphocytes
❏ E Gohn focus refers to involved regional lymph nodes
❏ F Gohn complex refers to the combination of the Gohn focus
 and involved regional lymph nodes
❏ G Gohn focus is usually subpleural in location

16. **Disseminated candidiasis**

❏ A usually produces positive blood cultures
❏ B commonly involves the eyes
❏ C is primarily treated with nystatin
❏ D is pre-disposed by long-term antibiotic treatment
❏ E has a similar prognosis in neutropenic patients

17. In the early assessment of severely injured patients

☐ A hypotension must be assumed to be hypovolaemic in origin until proven otherwise
☐ B loss of 50% or more of blood volume results in loss of consciousness
☐ C tourniquets are to be encouraged for control of limb blood loss
☐ D a high-riding prostate is a contraindication to urethral catheterization without a preceding urethrogram
☐ E neck wounds penetrating the platysma should be explored in the A&E Department

18. Recognised features of tension pneumothorax include

☐ A hypertension
☐ B absence of breath sounds on the affected side
☐ C hyper-resonance to percussion on the affected side
☐ D distended neck veins
☐ E tracheal deviation to the affected side

19. Following hepatobiliary trauma

☐ A Pringle's manoeuvre is used to prevent bile leakage from biliary tract
☐ B a ruptured gall bladder is usually treated by cholecystectomy
☐ C penetrating injuries have a higher mortality than those due to blunt injury
☐ D devitalised hepatic tissue should be excised
☐ E gallstone spillage is a major cause of late sepsis

20. Absolute contraindication(s) to diagnostic peritoneal lavage following abdominal trauma include

☐ A early pregnancy
☐ B indication for laparotomy
☐ C advanced cirrhosis
☐ D known gastrointestinal malignancy
☐ E previous abdominal operations

69

21. **In the investigation of thoracic and lumbar spine injuries, the following statements are true:**

❑ A thoracic spine fractures are rarely multiple
❑ B on plain X-ray, the width of the thoracic para-spinal line should normally be about one-third of the width of the descending thoracic aorta
❑ C simple wedge fractures of the lumbar spine can easily be differentiated from unstable or burst fractures on plain X-rays
❑ D AP, lateral and oblique views of the thoracic spine should be obtained in everyone with suspected thoracic spine injuries
❑ E on the AP lumbar spine view, the pedicles of L5 should be no further apart than the pedicles of L1

22. **In the treatment of spinal injuries**

❑ A iv naloxone has been shown to improve neurological recovery after spinal cord injury
❑ B iv methylprednisolone given during the first 24 hours significantly improves neurological recovery after spinal cord injury
❑ C unstable thoracic spine fractures require operation as soon as the patient is haemodynamically stable
❑ D fracture of the pedicles of the second cervical vertebra should initially be treated by in line traction
❑ E the initial neurological examination is a good predictor of prognosis

23. **Mammographic features suggestive of a malignant breast tumour include**

❑ A localised spiculated microcalcification of variable density
❑ B calcification of mammary blood vessels
❑ C diffuse coarse breast calcification
❑ D dense lesion of stellate appearance
❑ E nipple shadowing

24. **Agents clinically useful in the treatment of colorectal cancer include**

- A cyclophosphamide
- B 5-fluorouracil (5-FU)
- C vincristine
- D folinic acid (leucovorin)
- E cisplatin

25. **In the treatment of breast cancer, tamoxifen**

- A selectively binds to oestrogen receptors on breast cancer cells
- B is poorly tolerated by 40% of women
- C has no beneficial effect on pre-menopausal women
- D may cause vaginal bleeding
- E reduces the incidence of contralateral breast cancers

26. **Gastrointestinal consequences of major burns include**

- A splanchnic vasodilatation
- B acute gastric dilatation
- C Cushing's ulcers
- D paralytic ileus
- E terminal ileal lymphoid hyperplasia

27. **Relating to soft tissue coverage**

- A composite grafts include skin, subcutaneous tissue and cartilage
- B composite grafts maintain their own blood supply
- C human epithelial cells can be grown in tissue cultures to provide sheets for grafting
- D free flaps generally rely on blood supply from an artery of at least 3 mm in diameter
- E advancement flaps depend on skin laxity to provide excess tissue when separated from their underlying structures

28. **In coronary artery bypass surgery**

- ❑ A the patency rate of internal mammary artery grafts is approximately 90% at 10 years
- ❑ B the patency rate of vein grafts is approximately 80% at 10 years
- ❑ C the main risk factor predictive of outcome is left atrial function
- ❑ D early failure of the internal mammary graft function is usually due to a technical problem
- ❑ E long-term failure of vein grafts is due to suture fragmentation with embolization

29. **Laser surgery**

- ❑ A uses ultra-low dose irradiation to vaporise tissue
- ❑ B requires the use of non-reflective instruments
- ❑ C effects are independent of the type of tissue
- ❑ D effects vary according to the wavelength and power density used
- ❑ E is rarely precise

30. **After lateral hemi-section of the L5 segment of the spinal cord there is an ipsilateral**

- ❑ A loss of pain in the foot
- ❑ B loss of fine touch in the foot
- ❑ C loss of ankle jerk
- ❑ D wasting of the quadriceps muscle
- ❑ E Babinski sign

31. **The left brachiocephalic vein drains the**

- ❑ A cervical vertebrae
- ❑ B bronchi
- ❑ C intercostal spaces
- ❑ D thoracic duct
- ❑ E thyroid gland

32.   The middle lobe of the right lung

❏   A   is separated from the lower lobe by the transverse fissure
❏   B   may be auscultated at the 5ᵗʰ intercostal space posteriorly
❏   C   is indented by the right atrium
❏   D   has a diaphragmatic surface
❏   E   has three bronchopulmonary segments

33.   The diaphragm

❏   A   has a left crus attached to the L3 vertebra
❏   B   is pierced by the splanchnic nerves
❏   C   has an arterial supply from the abdominal aorta
❏   D   has a lateral arcuate ligament overlain by the kidney
❏   E   is related to the suprarenal glands

34.   The breast

❏   A   has an arterial supply from the axillary artery
❏   B   is drained by the internal thoracic vein
❏   C   has a nipple in the T3 dermatome
❏   D   drains 75% of its lymph via the axillary lymph nodes
❏   E   has a retro-mammary space over the pectoralis minor muscle

35.   Structures passing through the foramen magnum include

❏   A   medulla oblongata
❏   B   vertebral arteries
❏   C   spinal arteries
❏   D   vertebral veins
❏   E   dura mater

36.   Haemolytic anaemia

❏   A   is characteristically microcytic
❏   B   may lead to gallstones
❏   C   causes elevated urine urobilinogen levels
❏   D   causes elevated serum haptoglobin levels
❏   E   is associated with a conjugated hyperbilirubinaemia

37. **In the peri-operative management of patients with sickle cell disease**

❏ A antibiotic prophylaxis is only required in abdominal surgery
❏ B anti-thrombotic prophylaxis should be avoided
❏ C patients should be transfused to ensure a haemoglobin of > 14 g/dl
❏ D pre-operative fluids may help prevent vaso-occlusive events
❏ E exchange transfusion is only required for cardio-thoracic surgery

38. **Aspirin**

❏ A may be a useful anti-thrombotic following splenectomy
❏ B causes inhibition of cyclo-oxygenase for 24 hours
❏ C should be discontinued 48 hours before surgery to restore haemostasis
❏ D carries little risk of upper gastrointestinal bleeding

39. **Regarding coagulation factors**

❏ A the principle site of synthesis is the vascular endothelium
❏ B tissue factor expression by tumours may predispose to thrombosis
❏ C protein C has anti-coagulant activity
❏ D protein S has anti-coagulant activity
❏ E factor VII is a component of the extrinsic pathway

40. **Disseminated intravascular coagulation (DIC)**

❏ A is confirmed by elevated fibrinogen degradation products
❏ B produces a characteristic raised platelet count
❏ C is best managed with whole blood transfusion
❏ D is associated with increased fibrinolysis
❏ E may present with thrombosis

41.   Platelet transfusion should be administered

☐   A   only to patients with platelets of < 50 x 10⁹/l before
        ophthalmic surgery
☐   B   at a frequency of no more than two pools every 12 hours
☐   C   at least 36 hours pre-operatively to correct thrombocytopenia
☐   D   to all immune thrombocytopenia patients requiring elective
        splenectomy
☐   E   to all hospital patients with a platelet count of less than
        75 x 10⁹/l

**42.   In the assessment of a patient's need for peri-operative
        transfusion**

☐   A   cardiac output increases sharply when the haemoglobin falls
        below 10 g/dl
☐   B   blood volume is approximately 40 ml/kg in adults
☐   C   elderly patients with a haemoglobin of 4.8 g/dl should urgently
        receive six units of packed cells
☐   D   crystalloids are suitable as replacement for an acute bleeding
        in young patients with a loss of 15% intravascular blood
        volume
☐   E   men tolerate haemodilution better than women

**43.   Complications associated with massive blood transfusion
        include**

☐   A   hypokalaemia
☐   B   hypothermia
☐   C   disseminated intravascular coagulation
☐   D   thrombocytopenia
☐   E   eosinophilia

44.   Digoxin

☐   A   is used in the treatment of ventricular fibrillation
☐   B   potentiates the effect of warfarin
☐   C   has a high therapeutic index
☐   D   toxicity is potentiated by hypokalaemia
☐   E   usually converts atrial fibrillation into sinus rhythm

45.   In statistical analysis of clinical trial results

❑   A   the p-value is a probability with a value ranging from 0-100
❑   B   the p-value for significance is traditionally set at 0.01
❑   C   if one compares two means, the null hypothesis is that the two
            populations have different means
❑   D   a p-value of 0.001 is more significant than a p-value of 0.01

46.   Signs of acute haemolytic transfusion reaction include

❑   A   agitation
❑   B   pain at the cannula site
❑   C   hypertension
❑   D   coagulopathy
❑   E   oliguria

47.   Contraindications to colonoscopy include

❑   A   recent acute myocardial infarction
❑   B   known diverticular disease
❑   C   mild colitis
❑   D   peritonitis

SECTION 2 – EMQs

Theme: Classes of antibiotic

A Macrolide
B Quinolone
C Glycopeptide
D Monobactam

For each of the antibiotics listed below, select the correct antibiotic type from the list above. Each option may be used once, more than once, or not at all.

☐ 61. Aztreonam
☐ 62. Norfloxacin
☐ 63. Erythromycin
☐ 64. Vancomycin

Theme: Classification of organisms

A Fungal
B Protozoal
C Bacterial
D Viral

For each of the organisms listed below, select the correct group of organisms from the list above. Each option may be used once, more than once, or not at all.

☐ 65. Cryptosporidium
☐ 66. *Mycobacterium tuberculosis*
☐ 67. *Pneumocystis carinii*
☐ 68. *Cryptococcus neoformans*
☐ 69. Histoplasmosis
☐ 70. Aspergillus
☐ 71. *Nocardia asteroides*
☐ 72. *Listeria monocytogenes*

Theme: Arthropathy

A   Rheumatoid arthritis
B   Ankylosing spondylitis
C   Reiter's syndrome
D   Gout
E   Sarcoidosis
F   Calcium pyrophosphate deposition disease
G   Heberden's arthropathy
H   Psoriatic arthritis

For each patient with arthropathy, select the single most likely diagnosis from the list above. Each option may be used once, more than once or not at all.

☐   73.   A 20-year-old man with low back pain. He has bilateral sacroiliac joint tenderness and is tender over the insertion of his Achilles' tendons. He is otherwise well and has no antecedent history, although there is a history of similar problems in his father. HLA B27 antigen is positive.

☐   74.   A 50-year-old woman with carpal tunnel syndrome and an eight week history of metacarpophalangeal joint and ankle pain, which is worse in the mornings. She has a family history of joint problems. X-ray of her hands reveals periarticular erosions.

☐   75.   A 40-year-old man with arthritis of the distal interphalangeal joints of the hands and pitting of the nails.

☐   76.   A 30-year-old male presenting with pain and swelling of the left knee three weeks after an episode of non specific urethritis. He also complains of eye discomfort and dysuria.

Theme: Emergency resuscitation

A   Bag-Valve-Mask ventilation
B   Cricothyroidotomy
C   Guedel airway
D   Nasopharyngeal airway
E   Intravenous access (2 cannulae)
F   Chest drain insertion
G   Central line insertion
H   Arterial line insertion
I   Swan-Ganz catheter insertion

For each of the statements below, select the intervention you would perform next from the list above. Each option may be used once, more than once or not at all.

☐ 77. A 60-year-old man with severe abdominal pain, distension and diminished femoral pulses. BP 80/40 mmHg, pulse (brachial) 138/min. Pulse oximeter is not recording an oxygen saturation. He is breathing spontaneously and receiving high flow oxygen via a face mask with reservoir bag and is not cyanosed.

☐ 78. A patient admitted with crush injury to the chest. Saturations 85% on 15 L/min oxygen by face mask. The chest is dull to percussion and poor air entry right side of chest. Blood pressure 90 mmHg systolic, pulse 130/min, RR 35/min. Chest X-ray shows 'white-out' on the right side of chest with evidence of fluid accumulation.

Theme: Chest trauma

A Traumatic rupture of the thoracic aorta
B Traumatic myocardial contusion
C Cardiac tamponade
D Tension pneumothorax
E Massive haemothorax
F Flail chest

For each of the traumatic conditions listed below, select the most appropriate major clinical signs from the list above. Each option may be used once, more than once, or not at all.

☐ 79. Restricted chest wall movement and rib crepitus
☐ 80. Shock associated with unilateral absent breath sounds and dullness to percussion
☐ 81. Tracheal displacement to the opposite side
☐ 82. Muffled heart sounds and pulsus paradoxus
☐ 83. Pleural capping and tracheal deviation to the right
☐ 84. Depression of the left main bronchus and obliteration of the aorto-pulmonary window on CXR

Theme: Testicular tumours

A   Teratoma
B   Seminoma
C   Choriocarcinoma

For each of the statements below, select the most likely testicular tumour type from the list above. Each option may be used once, more than once, or not at all.

- ☐   85.   Secrete α fetoprotein (αFP) in approximately 70% of cases
- ☐   86.   Secrete βhCG in less than 10% of cases
- ☐   87.   Secrete either αFP or βhCG in about 90% of cases
- ☐   88.   Secrete βhCG in approximately 60% of cases
- ☐   89.   Almost always secrete βhCG

Theme: Chemotherapy regimens

A   Malignant carcinoid
B   Colorectal carcinoma
C   Testicular seminoma
D   Breast carcinoma

For each of the tumour scenarios listed below, select the most appropriate chemotherapeutic regimen from the list above. Each option may be used once, more than once, or not at all.

- ☐   90.   Combination 5-fluorouracil and folinic acid
- ☐   91.   Combination cyclophosphamide, methotrexate and 5-fluoro-uracil
- ☐   92.   Combination bleomycin, cisplatin and etoposide

Theme: Peripheral nerve anatomy

A Long thoracic
B Median
C Axillary
D Radial
E Musculocutaneous
F Ulnar
G Suprascapular
H Medial pectoral
I Thoracodorsal
J Upper subscapular

For each of the patients listed below, select the nerve most likely to be involved from the list above. Each option may be used once, more than once or not at all.

☐ 93. Whilst playing football, a young man dislocates his right shoulder. The dislocation is reduced soon after. Once the shoulder is pain free, he notices that he cannot carry weights with his right arm and is unable to raise his arm from his side for more than a few degrees. Neurological examination reveals loss of abduction and blunted sensation over the skin covering the lateral part of the deltoid muscle. All reflexes are normal.

☐ 94. After a radical mastectomy, a 40-year-old woman loses the ability to fold the right arm behind the back and reach up to the opposite scapula.

☐ 95. A 15-year-old boy riding in the passenger seat of a car escapes any apparent injury after a head-on collision, because he was wearing a seat belt. However, after the accident he found he was unable to raise the arm easily and has visited casualty twice with spontaneous dislocation of the shoulder.

☐ 96. A builder falls off scaffolding onto his right side fracturing his right humerus. Because of the patient's shocked state and the pain, only a limited neurological examination is possible which reveals an absence of the brachioradialis reflex, blunted cutaneous sensation over the first dorsal interosseous muscle, and wrist drop.

☐ 97. After a radical mastectomy, a 41-year-old woman is unable to push a loaded super-market trolley with her right arm. Her husband has noticed a deformity in her upper back on the right side which becomes more prominent when she pushes against resistance with the outstretched right arm.

Theme: Anatomy of the lungs and airways

A   Left main bronchus
B   Right main bronchus
C   Transthoracic plane
D   Left pulmonary artery
E   Left pulmonary vein
F   Trachea
G   Lobes of the lungs
H   Bronchial artery

For each of the statements below, select the most likely option from the list above. Each option may be used once, more than once or not at all.

☐   98.   Is separated from the arch of the aorta by the vagus nerve
☐   99.   Lies behind the left brachiocephalic vein
☐   100. Is the most anterior structure in the hilum
☐   101. Lies anterior to the oesophagus
☐   102. Bifurcates outside the lung

Theme: Anatomy of the brachial plexus and nerves of the upper arm

A   C5, C6, C7 roots of brachial plexus
B   C8, T1 roots of brachial plexus
C   Long thoracic nerve
D   Suprascapular nerve
E   Axillary nerve
F   Radial nerve
G   Ulnar nerve
H   Median nerve

For each patient with neurological abnormalities, select the single most likely site of nerve injury. Each option may be used once, more than once or not at all.

❑   103. A 3-day-old baby with a history of a difficult delivery followed by a floppy right arm. The arm is now held to the side, internally rotated and the forearm is pronated.
❑   104. A 28-year-old man has lost the use of his left hand since a motorcycle accident one week ago. Examination reveals a claw hand and left-sided Horner's syndrome.
❑   105. A 55-year-old woman complains of aching and weakness in her right arm following right mastectomy for breast carcinoma. Examination reveals winging of the right scapula on pressing against a wall.
❑   106. A 20-year-old man following a anterior dislocation of his right shoulder playing rugby has loss of abduction of the shoulder.
❑   107. A 43-year-old man presents with a weak left arm since a drinking binge. He is unable to extend his wrist or elbow.

Theme: Peripheral nerves of the upper limb

A Radial nerve
B Median nerve
C Ulnar nerve
D Posterior interosseous nerve
E Anterior interosseous nerve
F Superficial branch of ulnar nerve
G Deep branch of ulnar nerve

For each patient with nerve compression symptoms, select the nerve most likely to be involved. Each option may be used once, more than once or not at all.

☐ 108. A 23-year-old long distance cyclist notices difficulty in writing after a race. There is weakness of finger adduction and abduction but normal sensation in the hand. Froment's sign is positive.

☐ 109. A 30-year-old right-handed lady complains of pain and clumsiness after playing the piano. She has weak thumb and index finger flexion, but no sensory deficit.

☐ 110. An 18-year-old weight lifter develops paraesthesia in the ulnar two digits of his right hand. On examination, there is sensory loss in the little and ring fingers, but no motor loss.

Theme: Interpretation of the laboratory features of acquired
         coagulation disorders

A   Heparin therapy
B   Established warfarin therapy
C   Aspirin therapy
D   Hepatic insufficiency
E   Acquired von Willebrand's disease

For each set of results below, select the most likely cause for the
abnormalities from the list of options above. Each option may be used
once, more than once or not at all.

Normal ranges:
    Prothrombin time (PT)   12–16 s
    Activated partial thromboplastin time (APTT)   26–38 s
    Thrombin time (TT)   11–15 s
    Fibrinogen (FIB)   1.5–4.5 g/dl

❑   111. PT 28   APTT 56   TT 22   FIB 2.5
❑   112. PT 14   APTT 58   TT 11   FIB 3.1
❑   113. PT 16   APTT 52   TT 124   FIB 1.9
❑   114. PT 15   APTT 37   TT 12   FIB 2.9
❑   115. PT 24   APTT 49   TT 28   FIB 0.9

Theme: Diagnosis of acute blood transfusion reactions

A   Non-haemolytic febrile transfusion reaction
B   Delayed haemolytic transfusion reaction
C   Anaphylactic reaction
D   Urticarial reaction
E   Haemolytic reaction not due to ABO incompatibility
F   Acute haemolytic transfusion reaction

For each of the following clinical scenarios following blood transfusion, select the most likely diagnosis from the list of options above. Each option may be used once, more than once or not at all.

☐ 116. A 32-year-old man receiving a fresh frozen plasma infusion develops sudden onset wheezing, tachypnoea and tachycardia. His clinical course rapidly deteriorates and he becomes cyanosed and hypotensive.

☐ 117. A 74-year-old man develops nausea and fever one hour after a red cell transfusion. The next day he is noted to be jaundiced and has failed to achieve his expected haemoglobin.

☐ 118. A 28-year-old multi-parous woman develops a headache and chills one hour after starting a red cell transfusion. She is noted to be febrile. Her symptoms rapidly settle when she is given paracetamol and the transfusion is slowed down.

END OF CORE PAPER 4

Time allowed: 2 hours
Indicate your answers in the spaces provided

Section 1 – MCQs

1. **Physiological responses to loss of circulating blood volume include**

   ❏ A peripheral venular vasoconstriction
   ❏ B peripheral arteriolar vasoconstriction
   ❏ C reduced resistance to blood flow
   ❏ D transcapillary refilling
   ❏ E haemoconcentration
   ❏ F tachycardia

2. **Recognised complications of central venous line insertion include**

   ❏ A arterial air embolism
   ❏ B haemorrhage
   ❏ C pneumothorax
   ❏ D chylothorax
   ❏ E venous air embolism

3. **General host factors predisposing to wound infection include**

   ❏ A hypoxia
   ❏ B pyrexia
   ❏ C jaundice
   ❏ D hypercalcaemia
   ❏ E anaemia

4. **Cardiopulmonary bypass**

   ❏ A is often associated with thrombocytosis
   ❏ B is often associated with platelet dysfunction
   ❏ C is usually combined with induced hyperthermia
   ❏ D does not affect coagulation factor levels
   ❏ E vitamin K is administered at the end of bypass to neutralise remaining circulating heparin

5. **Features of Adult Respiratory Distress Syndrome (ARDS) include**

    ☐ A   interstitial and alveolar oedema
    ☐ B   granulomata
    ☐ C   hyaline membrane formation
    ☐ D   glandular hyperplasia
    ☐ E   interstitial fibrosis

6. **The following suggest that respiratory failure is chronic rather than acute:**

    ☐ A   bicarbonate of 39 mmol/l
    ☐ B PaO_2 of 9 kPa
    ☐ C PaO_2 of 7 kPa
    ☐ D   arterial pH of 7.2
    ☐ E   the presence of a hypoxic respiratory drive

7. **Central venous pressure (CVP)**

    ☐ A   is affected by posture
    ☐ B   is elevated in right ventricular failure
    ☐ C   is normal in septic shock
    ☐ D   accurately reflects cardiac output
    ☐ E   is raised in hypertension

8. **Acute renal failure**

    ☐ A   is due to nephrotoxic drugs in 50% cases
    ☐ B   occurs in approximately 30% of critically ill patients
    ☐ C   may produce little histological change
    ☐ D   is usually the result of damage to the proximal tubule
    ☐ E   carries an overall mortality rate of 10%

9. **Penetrating hepatic trauma**

☐ A   may be managed conservatively
☐ B   may cause haemobilia
☐ C   is usually fatal
☐ D   causing excessive bleeding is best controlled by packing gauze swabs into the hepatic defect
☐ E   causing excessive bleeding may be controlled by Pringle's manoeuvre

10. **'Open' or 'sucking' pneumothorax**

☐ A   results from a chest wall defect which remains open
☐ B   causes air to pass preferentially through the chest wall with each respiratory effort
☐ C   impairs gaseous exchange but not ventilation
☐ D   is treated acutely by sealing the chest wall defect completely
☐ E   defects usually require definitive surgical closure

11. **Flail chest**

☐ A   usually results from trauma associated with multiple rib fractures
☐ B   produces ventilatory problems due to loss of local chest wall movement
☐ C   often requires artificial ventilation to prevent hypoxia
☐ D   patients should be monitored in an intensive therapy unit

12. **In the investigation of acute cervical spine injuries**

☐ A   a good quality lateral cervical spine film will identify approximately 75% of significant cervical spine injuries in adults
☐ B   an acceptable lateral cervical spine X-ray should include the upper border of T1
☐ C   normal AP, lateral and odontoid peg views effectively exclude significant cervical spine injury
☐ D   flexion and extension X-ray views are the best method of excluding ligamentous injury
☐ E   spinal cord injury without radiological abnormality is commoner in children than in adults.

13.   The following are typical features of an acute extradural
        haematoma on CT scan:

❑   A   crescent shaped haematoma
❑   B   haematoma crossing the suture line
❑   C   haematoma crossing the midline
❑   D   associated skull fracture
❑   E   decreased attenuation of the haematoma

14.   Major incidence planning

❑   A   should involve high level officials of the local police, fire and
        ambulance services
❑   B   should be recorded and tested
❑   C   requires adequate provision of communication facilities
❑   D   should involve evacuation of patients already hospitalised for
        conditions unrelated to the disaster
❑   E   should be co-ordinated by the most senior surgical registrar in
        the hospital

15.   Early features of acute compartment syndrome include

❑   A   loss of distal pulses
❑   B   excessive pain
❑   C   pain on passive movement
❑   D   paraesthesia
❑   E   pallor

16.   In a multi-trauma patient

❑   A   the maximum rate of fluid administration is determined by the
        internal diameter
❑   B   a minimum of four large gauge venflons should be inserted
❑   C   initial fluid replacement should be with blood
❑   D   hypovolaemic shock is treated with vasopressive agents
❑   E   hypothermia may produce cardiac dysrhythmias

17.   Medications which should be continued until the morning of the operation include

❑ A   anti-hypertensive drugs
❑ B   chlorpropamide
❑ C   oral nitrates
❑ D   monoamine oxidase inhibitors (MAOIs)
❑ E   carbamazepine

18.   Prognosis of malignant melanoma is related to

❑ A   clinical stage
❑ B   Breslow tumour thickness
❑ C   sex
❑ D   ulceration
❑ E   degree of melanosis

19.   Which of the following have malignant potential:

❑ A   Bowen's disease
❑ B   solar keratosis
❑ C   keratoacanthoma
❑ D   Spitz naevus
❑ E   molluscum contagiosum
❑ F   basal cell papilloma

20.   Cutaneous squamous cell carcinomas

❑ A   are associated with xeroderma pigmentosa
❑ B   may complicate long-standing venous ulceration
❑ C   may regress to produce Bowen's disease
❑ D   have an increased incidence in renal transplant recipients
❑ E   metastasise to lymph nodes in approximately 15% of cases
❑ F   behave more aggressively when found on the vulva

21.   Staging of malignant tumours

❑ A   helps one to prognosticate
❑ B   includes details of loco-regional and distant sites
❑ C   can be made solely on the basis of a histological specimen
         alone
❑ D   may be altered by response to irradiation treatment
❑ E   takes into account the local anatomy for individual primary
         tumour sites

22.   Colorectal carcinoma

❑ A   is thought to arise from pre-existing polyps in 25% of cases
❑ B   is more common following ureterosigmoidostomy
❑ C   is associated with abnormalities of chromosome 17
❑ D   breaching the bowel wall and spreading into the perirectal
         tissues is classified as Duke's C
❑ E   usually spreads in a longitudinal manner within the wall of the
         bowel

23.   Malignant testicular tumours

❑ A   are mostly germ-cell tumours
❑ B   have a peak incidence between 20–40 years of age
❑ C   are falling in incidence
❑ D   teratomas are more radiosensitive than seminomas
❑ E   seminomas have a greater metastatic potential and a worse
         prognosis than teratomas
❑ F   seminomas tend to present at an earlier age than teratomas

24.   Mammographic screening for breast cancer

❑ A   has been shown to reduce deaths from breast cancer by up to
         30%
❑ B   detects malignant lesions in 4 per 1000 patients
❑ C   detects malignant lesions in 4 per 1000 cases in patients aged
         56–64 years at subsequent screens
❑ D   is conducted biennially
❑ E   is cost-effective in patients aged 30 years and over

25.   Phylloides tumours (cystosarcoma phylloides) of the breast

☐ A   are mostly malignant
☐ B   have a fleshy and lobulated appearance when cut
☐ C   contain a benign epithelial component
☐ D   commonly spread to regional nodes
☐ E   may recur after resection

26.   Adjuvant chemotherapy for breast cancer

☐ A   single agent chemotherapy has a greater beneficial effect on survival than combination chemotherapy
☐ B   is most commonly given by intermittent injection
☐ C   is the treatment of choice for metastases
☐ D   has little role in the treatment of inflammatory cancers
☐ E   has a clinical response limited to pre-menopausal women

27.   The following are considered to be pre-malignant conditions:

☐ A   Barrett's oesophagus
☐ B   Paget's disease of the breast
☐ C   Peutz-Jeghers syndrome
☐ D   balanitis xerotica obliterans
☐ E   Familial Adenomatous Polyposis

28.   In the management of breast cysts

☐ A   aspiration usually reveals blood-stained fluid
☐ B   simple cysts should have no residual lump following aspiration
☐ C   recurrent cysts may be repeatedly aspirated without risk of missing an underlying malignancy
☐ D   90% will not recur following aspiration
☐ E   blood-stained aspiration fluid is pathognomonic of an underlying duct papilloma

29. **Split skin grafting (SSG) of clean, granulating wounds is usually contraindicated in the presence of**

- ❏ A MRSA
- ❏ B Pseudomonas
- ❏ C *Staphylococcus epidermidis*
- ❏ D *Beta-haemolytic streptococci*
- ❏ E Klebsiella

30. **Viral hepatitis**

- ❏ A hepatitis A is a RNA virus
- ❏ B hepatitis B is a RNA virus
- ❏ C hepatitis A has an incubation period of 2–5 days
- ❏ D hepatitis A rarely causes fulminant hepatitis
- ❏ E hepatitis A may give rise to a carrier state

31. **The risk of overwhelming post-splenectomy sepsis may be reduced by**

- ❏ A HiB vaccination
- ❏ B hepatitis B vaccination
- ❏ C poliomyelitis vaccination
- ❏ D prophylactic metronidazole
- ❏ E pneumococcal vaccination

32. **Diathermy**

- ❏ A uses a low current density for thermocautery
- ❏ B using a high frequency alternating current has less chance of causing ventricular fibrillation
- ❏ C may cause accidental burns if the patient is near but not touching earth
- ❏ D belongs to Class 3 of the International Electrotechnical Commission Standards
- ❏ E cannot be used in a patient with a pacemaker

33. **Spinal hemi-section at the lower level of the C5 cord segment results in ipsilateral loss of**

☐ A   diaphragmatic movement
☐ B   shoulder shrugging movements
☐ C   pain and temperature sensation below the lesion
☐ D   touch below the lesion
☐ E   cutaneous sensation over the clavicle

34. **The transthoracic plane (of Louis) intersects the**

☐ A   azygos vein
☐ B   right recurrent laryngeal nerve
☐ C   ligamentum venosum
☐ D   bifurcation of the pulmonary trunk
☐ E   upper border of the aortic arch

35. **Bronchial metastases enlarging at the hilum of the left lung may cause**

☐ A   the dome of the diaphragm to be depressed on X-ray
☐ B   laryngeal stridor
☐ C   paraesthesia over the left shoulder
☐ D   enlargement of the infraclavicular lymph nodes
☐ E   dyspnoea

36. **Signs of L5 nerve root compression include**

☐ A   weakness of the extensor hallucis longus
☐ B   allodynia in the L5 dermatome
☐ C   weakness of ankle dorsiflexion
☐ D   wasting of extensor digitorum brevis
☐ E   loss of sensation in the S1 dermatome

37. **The right atrium**

- [ ] A   forms the right border of the heart
- [ ] B   lies in front of the left atrium
- [ ] C   has the coronary sinus opening above the septal cusp of the tricuspid valve
- [ ] D   has a posterior wall formed by the interatrial septum
- [ ] E   has the sinoatrial node medial to the sulcus terminalis

38. **The treatment of acute haemolytic transfusion reaction includes**

- [ ] A   removing the iv cannula from the patient
- [ ] B   fluid restriction to avoid pulmonary oedema
- [ ] C   frusemide
- [ ] D   1 litre 20% mannitol
- [ ] E   insertion of a central line in an oliguric patient

39. **The prothrombin time**

- [ ] A   measures the activity of the extrinsic coagulation pathway
- [ ] B   is not usually prolonged in liver disease
- [ ] C   is prolonged in haemophilia A
- [ ] D   can be expressed as the INR when monitoring warfarin dosage
- [ ] E   is prolonged in vitamin K malabsorption

40. **Intravascular haemolysis**

- [ ] A   seldom occurs after ABO mis-matched blood transfusion
- [ ] B   may occur after burns
- [ ] C   is common in autoimmune haemolytic anaemia
- [ ] D   may occur in disseminated intravascular coagulation
- [ ] E   may occur after mitral valve replacement

41.   With regards to the complications of anticoagulant therapy

☐ A   heparin should be urgently withdrawn in the event of thrombocytopenia
☐ B   skin necrosis is a recognised hazard
☐ C   osteoporosis may complicate long-term warfarin therapy
☐ D   warfarin should be avoided in pregnancy
☐ E   low molecular weight heparins are associated with fewer bleeding complications than unfractionated heparin

42.   Platelet count

☐ A   of < 50 x 10^9/l is likely to cause spontaneous bleeding of the colon
☐ B   may be elevated in patients with an adenocarcinoma
☐ C   characteristically falls after splenectomy
☐ D   may be influenced by phlebotomy technique
☐ E   may be decreased in patients with an adenocarcinoma of the colon

43.   Autologous blood transfusion

☐ A   eliminates the risk of transmitted infection transmission
☐ B   is useful for Jehovah's Witness patients
☐ C   must undergo ABO and Rhesus D typing
☐ D   can supply up to 10 units of red cells
☐ E   eliminates the need for donor blood

44.   The following are recognised sequelae of massive blood transfusion:

☐ A   hyperkalaemia
☐ B   hypocalcaemia
☐ C   dilutional thrombocytopenia
☐ D   adult respiratory distress syndrome
☐ E   hyperthermia

45.   Which of the following are cryoprecipitates:

- ❑ A   factor VI
- ❑ B   platelets
- ❑ C   fibrinogen
- ❑ D   von Willebrand factor
- ❑ E   fresh frozen plasma

46.   Iron deficiency anaemia may be associated with

- ❑ A   a raised serum ferritin
- ❑ B   dysphagia
- ❑ C   a reduced serum iron binding capacity
- ❑ D   pica
- ❑ E   peripheral neuropathy

47.   In the setting of clinical trials

- ❑ A   single blinding refers to the patient not knowing which treatment he/she has received
- ❑ B   double blinding refers to both the patient and their family not knowing which treatment the patient has received
- ❑ C   randomisation refers to a selection process in which treatment options are decided for individual patients
- ❑ D   a control group is a group of observers that oversees the conduction of a clinical trial
- ❑ E   using historical controls provides a more reliable group for comparison than a group randomised to control

SECTION 2 – EMQs

Theme: Cardiorespiratory arrest

A Commence CPR, intubate, iv access, adrenaline (epinephrine), look for tension pneumothorax, cardiac tamponade, hypovolaemia and other reasons for EMD.

B CPR – defibrillate as soon as possible, initially 200 J followed by a further 200 J, then 360 if unresponsive

C CPR – iv access, intravenous calcium and adrenaline (epinephrine)

D Commence CPR, intubate, iv access, adrenaline (epinephrine), consider atropine

E Start CPR, give DC shock at 200 J then if no response give intracardiac adrenaline (epinephrine)

F Give intravenous fluids, if no response, 1 mg of adrenaline (epinephrine).

G Precordial thump, if no success, immediate defibrillation, initially with 200 J shock

H Ventilate with bag and mask ventilation, intubate, iv access, review

I Check for pulse, rhythm, if none, start CPR and tilt patient on to left side. Gain iv access and intubate (if possible).

For each of the patients listed below, choose the ERC recommended treatment of choice from the list above. Each option may be used once, more than once or not at all.

61. 56-year-old male monitored in Coronary Care Unit, witnessed ventricular fibrillation arrest
62. 28-year-old female in EMD after an RTA
63. 72-year-old male post-op right inguinal hernia repair, asystole
64. 7-year-old male asthmatic – respiratory arrest
65. 24-year-old female collapsed after massive ante-partum haemorrhage
66. 62-year-old male found following cardiopulmonary arrest – ventricular tachycardia, no pulse

Theme: Investigations for DVT

A Clinical examination
B Doppler ultrasound (duplex)
C Impedance plethysmography
D Phlebography
E Radioiodine-labelled fibrinogen scan

For each of the statements below, select the correct investigation from the list of options above. Each option may be used once, more than once, or not at all.

- ❑ 67. Indicates the extent and degree of fixity of thrombus
- ❑ 68. Is contraindicated in the presence of severe peripheral vascular disease
- ❑ 69. Has a 50% false-positive rate
- ❑ 70. Lower limb incisions can give false-positives
- ❑ 71. Has a risk of inducing hepatitis

Theme: Benign lesions of skin and lymphatics

A Pilomatrixoma
B Cylindroma
C Ganglion
D Cystic hygroma
E Syringoma

For each tissue of origin listed below, select the correct benign lesion from the list above. Each option may be used once, more than once, or not at all.

- ❑ 72. Lymphatic channels
- ❑ 73. Apocrine gland
- ❑ 74. Synovial sheath
- ❑ 75. Eccrine gland
- ❑ 76. Hair follicle

Theme: Mode of tumour spread

A Local invasion
B Blood-borne spread
C Trans-coelomic spread
D Lymphatic spread

For each of the tumours below, select the predominant mode of spread from the list above. Each option may be used once, more than once, or not at all.

☐ 77. Seminoma of the testis
☐ 78. Cutaneous basal cell carcinoma
☐ 79. Papillary thyroid carcinoma
☐ 80. Follicular thyroid carcinoma
☐ 81. Ovarian carcinoma

Theme: Thyroid cancer

A Papillary carcinoma
B Follicular carcinoma
C Medullary cell carcinoma
D Anaplastic carcinoma
E Lymphoma
F Thyroid secondaries from another primary organ

For each of the statements below, select the correct thyroid carcinoma from the list above. Each option may be used once, more than once, or not at all.

☐ 82. Early haematogenous and lymphatic spread
☐ 83. Is usually very radiosensitive
☐ 84. Accounts for 60% of thyroid carcinoma cases
☐ 85. Is derived from parafollicular C cells
☐ 86. Commonly metastasises to bone and lung but lymphatic spread is unusual

Theme: Bone and joint sepsis

A   *Mycobacterium tuberculosis*
B   *Staphylococcus aureus*
C   *Haemophilus influenzae*
D   Gonococcus
E   *Salmonella typhi*
F   β-haemolytic streptococcus
G   *Clostridium perfringens*
H   *Clostridium difficile*

For each clinical situation below, select the organism that is the most likely cause of the pathology from the list above. Each option may be used once, more than once or not at all.

□   87.   A 20-year-old man with a history of drug abuse, presents with soft tissue swelling, tenderness and erythema of the left forearm. There are multiple tender lymph nodes in the axilla.

□   88.   A child with known sickle cell disease presents with a three day history of increasing pain and swelling over the distal humerus where there is exquisite tenderness. She is pyrexial, has a raised ESR and WCC. Her X-ray shows changes suggestive of a bone infarct.

□   89.   A patient known to have AIDS and with a low CD4 count, presents with a chronically painful and swollen ankle which has been discharging milky fluid via two sinuses for the past two weeks. The ankle is not particularly hot or inflamed.

□   90.   Ella aged two presents with a reluctance to walk following her first day back at play-group after recovering from a nasty chesty cold. All movements of her left hip are painful.

□   91.   A film producer working in a small African town fell backwards into a sewage pit and sustained an open fracture dislocation of his ankle. It was reduced in the township and placed in a temporary splint. He elected to fly home for treatment. On arrival in Casualty 36 hours later he was septic with an acutely painful, swollen and red lower limb.

Theme: Trauma

A Flail chest
B Fracture of C3
C Basal skull fracture
D Fractured 1st rib
E Ruptured diaphragm
F Massive haemothorax
G Jefferson's fracture
H Cardiac tamponade
I Hangman's fracture

For each of the statements in the list below, select the most appropriate option from the list above. Each option may be used once, more than once or not at all.

☐ 92. Gas bubble seen above diaphragm on CXR
☐ 93. Battle's sign
☐ 94. Paradoxical breathing associated with pulmonary contusions
☐ 95. Ring blow-out of C1
☐ 96. Associated with major vessel injury
☐ 97. Paralysis of the phrenic nerve

Theme: Pelvic fracture

A Stable pelvic fracture
B Rotationally unstable, vertically stable pelvic fracture
C Rotationally unstable, vertically unstable pelvic fracture

For each of the pelvic injuries below, select the correct classification of pelvic fracture from the list above. Each option may be used once, more than once, or not at all.

☐ 98. Lateral compression fracture
☐ 99. Open book fracture
☐ 100. Vertical shear injuries
☐ 101. Isolated iliac wing fracture
☐ 102. Isolated pubic ramus fracture

Theme: Burns

A   1%
B   4.5%
C   7%
D   9%
E   14%
F   18%

For each of the statements below regarding adult cutaneous burns, select the correct percentage of the total body surface area from the list above. Each option may be used once, more than once, or not at all.

- ☐ 103. Burns to all the head and neck
- ☐ 104. Burns to all the anterior trunk (chest/abdomen)
- ☐ 105. Burns to all the male genitals
- ☐ 106. Burns to all the posterior trunk (upper and lower back)
- ☐ 107. Burns to the whole anterior aspect of one leg
- ☐ 108. Burns to the whole anterior aspect of one arm
- ☐ 109. Burns to the whole posterior aspect of both legs

Theme: Multiple Endocrine Neoplasia syndromes

A   Multiple Endocrine Neoplasia I
B   Multiple Endocrine Neoplasia IIA
C   Multiple Endocrine Neoplasia IIB

For each option given below, select the most likely MEN syndrome from the list above. Each option may be used once, more than once, or not at all.

- ☐ 110. Submucosal neuromas
- ☐ 111. Pancreatic islet cell adenomas
- ☐ 112. Marfanoid appearance
- ☐ 113. Pituitary hyperplasia

Theme: **Anatomy of the brachial plexus**

A   C7 root
B   Posterior cord
C   Upper trunk
D   Middle trunk
E   C6 root
F   Medial cord
G   Median nerve
H   Anterior divisions

For each of the statements below, select the most likely option from the list below. Each option may be used once, more than once or not at all.

☐   114. Is formed by branches from two different cords
☐   115. Gives off the suprascapular nerve
☐   116. Has no contribution from anterior divisions
☐   117. Is formed from a single anterior division
☐   118. Is a direct continuation of the C7 root
☐   119. Innervates the entire flexor compartment of the upper limb
☐   120. Receives a grey ramus from the inferior cervical (or stellate) sympathetic ganglion
☐   121. Contributes a branch to the long thoracic nerve (of Bell)

Theme: Interpretation of haematinic results

A   Previous total gastrectomy
B   Carcinoma of the rectum
C   Previous massive small bowel resection
D   Extensive jejunal diverticula
E   Chronic haemorrhagic gastritis with acute urinary tract infection

For each of the sets of results below, select the most likely diagnosis from the list of options above. Each option may be used once only, more than once or not at all.

Normal ranges:

Ferritin	15–250 µg/l
Total iron binding capacity (TIBC)	250–400 µg/l
Serum B_{12}	150–900 ng/L
Serum folate	4–20 µg/l

- [ ] 122. Hb 6.6 g/dl   MCV 72 fl   Ferritin 12   TIBC 787
- [ ] 123. Hb 9.2g/dl   MCV 115 fl   Ferritin 82 B_{12} 112   Folate 105
- [ ] 124. Hb 10.7 g/dl   MCV 91 fl   Ferritin 12 B_{12} 155   Folate 3
- [ ] 125. Hb 4.8 g/dl   MCV 111 fl   Ferritin 72 B_{12} 30   Folate 47
- [ ] 126. Hb 10.0 g/dl   MCV 71 fl   Ferritin 345   TIBC 380

Theme: Treatment of haemostatic disorders

A   Vitamin K and fresh frozen plasma
B   Cryoprecipitate and fresh frozen plasma
C   Recombinant factor VIII concentrate
D   Intermediate purity factor VIII concentrate
E   Platelets, cryoprecipitate and fresh frozen plasma

For each of the scenarios below, select the most appropriate treatment from the list of options above. Each option may be used once, more than once or not at all.

Normal ranges:
Prothrombin time (PT)	12–16 s
Activated partial thromboplastin time (APTT)	26–38 s
Platelet count (Plt)	150–400 x 10^9/l
Fibrinogen (FIB)	2–4 g/dl x 10^9/l
Factor VIII	50–150 iu/ml
von Willebrand factor	50–150 iu/ml

☐   127. A 42-year-old man is admitted with acute cholecystitis. Despite antibiotic treatment he becomes hypotensive, oliguric and hypoxic. His coagulation screen shows PT 28 s, APTT 73 s, FIB 0.2 g/dl and Plt 59 x10^9/l.

☐   128. A 39-year-old woman is admitted for a subtotal thyroidectomy. She has a history of easy bruising and gum bleeding. There is a similar family history. Her coagulation tests show PT 14 s, APTT 64 s, Factor VIII 5 iu/ml, von Willebrand factor 6 iu/ml.

☐   129. A 43-year-old man on warfarin for a prosthetic mitral valve presents with confusion following a fall. There is radiographic evidence of an acute subdural haematoma that requires urgent surgical drainage. His PT is 89 s.

END OF CORE PAPER 5

CORE PAPER 1
SECTION 1 – MCQS

1.   Wound healing   Answers: B C
Wounds of the skin, subcutaneous tissues, muscle, fascia and tendon only ever regain 80–90% of their pre-injury strength. The development of wound strength is dependent on the type of collagen produced. In the early phase of wound healing, type III collagen is produced which is weaker than the later appearing type I collagen (maturation stage). The process of skin healing includes a lag phase lasting 1–2 weeks following injury, followed by a proliferative phase lasting 2–12 weeks, and finally a scar maturation phase lasting months to years.

2.   Metabolic responses to surgery   Answers: A D E
Surgery leads to a complex metabolic response mediated by neural and hormonal reflexes. These include increased secretion of aldosterone, ADH, catecholamines, glucagon, cortisol, thyroxine, and growth hormone. ADH increases urinary potassium excretion and reduces sodium and water excretion. Catecholamines increase skeletal muscle breakdown, urinary nitrogen excretion, lipolysis, and circulating free fatty acids (FFAs), and reduce protein anabolism. Glucagon, cortisol, thyroxine, and growth hormone increase basal metabolic rate and blood glucose through glycogenolysis and gluconeogenesis, so leading to impaired glucose tolerance.

3.   Antibiotic prophylaxis   Answers: B C D
From prospective randomised controlled trials, antibiotic prophylaxis in surgery has been established to be of proven benefit. Infection is only prevented when antibiotics are given just prior to or at the time of surgery. With the exception of prolonged operations, single dose prophylaxis is effective in most clinical situations. A further dose is given if the operation lasts longer than four hours. Full doses of the correct antibiotics should be given (ones with proven efficacy to prevent wound infection).

4.   Oesophageal cancer   Answers: A C
Oesophageal cancer has a very poor prognosis, with most patients incurable at diagnosis. The overall 1-year survival is about 30%, and the overall 5-year survival is about 5–10%. It is associated with prominent lymphatic permeation so producing microscopic metastases beyond the macroscopic limits of the tumour. Stenting of upper-third tumours is poorly tolerated by patients and may also compromise the airway. β naphthylamine increases the risk of developing bladder cancer.

5.   **Radiotherapy for breast cancer**   Answers: B D

Radiotherapy has never been shown to improve overall survival from breast cancer, and in fact some trials have shown increased death rates from cardiovascular disease. However, post-op radiotherapy clearly reduces local recurrence rates following conservative breast surgery. There is a high risk of severe arm lymphoedema following combined axillary clearance and radiotherapy. Radiotherapy should not be applied to the axilla after a complete lymph node clearance but may be given if the nodes have been sampled and are positive for tumour. A radiotherapy boost is often added to the internal mammary chain lymph nodes for medial tumours.

6.   **Surgery for breast cancer**   Answers: A C E

Relative indications for conservative breast excision rather than mastectomy for breast cancer include localised disease, smaller tumours, larger breasts, impalpable disease, and patient choice. Oestrogen receptor and menopausal status should not influence the type of surgery.

7.   **Bone tumours**   Answers: A B

Malignant primary bone tumours are rare, but benign tumours such as osteomas are more common. The commonest bone tumour is a metastasis from a primary malignant tumour at another site. Ewing's sarcoma has an overall poor prognosis. Benign bone tumours tend to occur in adolescents and young adults. Primary malignant bone tumours are often very aggressive and tend to occur in adolescents and young adults. There is often a characteristic history of pain. These lesions have ill-defined margins on X-ray (Codman's triangle, sun-ray spicules).

8.   **Male breast carcinoma**   Answers: A D E

Male breast cancer is 100 times less common than the female variety. The aetiology is unknown but there is an increased incidence in Klinefelter's syndrome. Male breast carcinoma tends to present at a later stage than female breast carcinoma. The preferred surgical treatment is mastectomy.

9.   **HNPCC**   Answers: B C

HNPCC is associated with an early age of onset of colorectal cancers, with an increased incidence of both proximal bowel cancers and endometrial cancers compared to the general population. HNPCC is more commonly of the mucinous form, and is less well-differentiated compared to colonic carcinomas in the general population. Despite this, the 5-year survival for HNPCC colonic cancers compared to those of the general population is better.

10.   Screening programmes   **Answers: A D E**

Results of screening programmes for cancer are limited by selection, length and lead time bias. Selection bias arises from the tendency of people who enrol on screening programmes to be more health conscious and are therefore atypical of the general population. Length bias is the tendency for screening to detect a disproportionate number of cancers which are slow growing and have a better prognosis anyway. Lead-time bias is the phenomenon that screening advances the date at which diagnosis is made. This, therefore, lengthens the survival time without necessarily altering the date of death.

11.   Third space fluid loss   **Answers: A B C**

Third space loss is internal and is the temporary loss of extracellular fluid into a space, which does not participate in the transport of nutrients or waste products. In moderately large operations such as cholecystectomy, loss would be approximately 3 ml/kg/hr. In more major operations such as aortic aneurysm repair, third space fluid loss could initially be 10–20 ml/kg/hr. Dextrose saline is hypotonic. When dextrose is metabolised, it increases free water content and so leads to hypo-natraemia. Balanced salt solutions should be used to replace third space losses. Transcellular losses which one might be able to measure include ascites, pleural effusions and intra-intestinal losses.

12.   Epidural anaesthesia   **Answers: A C D**

Epidural blockade involves entering the epidural space with a needle, introducing a catheter and then infusing local anaesthetic. The dura may be inadvertently punctured by the needle or catheter resulting in headache. The local anaesthetic prevents transmission in the sensory, motor and autonomic sympathetic nerve fibres. A sympathetic blockade would cause hypotension and bradycardia, a motor blockade would cause hypoventilation and urinary retention.

13.   Bupivacaine   **Answer: D**

Local anaesthetics are made heavy by preparation in 8% dextrose so that they are hyperbaric in the cerebro-spinal fluid and so have a predictable spread. 0.5% bupivacaine is equivalent to 0.5 g in 100 ml, so 10 ml contains 50 mg. 1 in 200,000 adrenaline is equivalent to 1 g in 200,000 ml, so 10 ml contains 50 micrograms. The preparation here is unsuitable for intravenous injection, as bupivacaine would cause severe dysrhythmias.

14.   Dopexamine   **Answers: B C D**
Dopexamine is a dopaminergic agonist with β– and no α-adrenergic actions. Dopexamine has little effect on the mean arterial pressure. It increases the cardiac index by reducing systemic vascular resistance. These haemodynamic effects cause both natriuretic and diuretic actions. A clear renoprotective role for dopexamine has yet to be shown.

15.   Elective cholecystectomy   **Answer: A E**
A 50-year-old diabetic is at risk of cardiac disease and so U&E, FBC, CXR and ECG are all justified. The best assessment of diabetic control is glycosylated haemoglobin (HbA$_{1c}$). His blood glucose may be controlled perioperatively by the Alberti regimen which comprises a simultaneous infusion of 5% dextrose containing potassium chloride and intravenous insulin. The resulting blood sugar may be measured accurately by bedside tests but the laboratory is required for measurement of serum potassium concentration.

16.   MODS   **Answer: C**
MODS is dysfunction of more than one organ, requiring intervention to maintain homeostasis. The overall prognosis of established MODS is very poor despite aggressive treatment. To optimise chances of recovery, the underlying problem should be corrected and supportive therapy (including nutrition) instituted. There is presently no evidence to show that anti-endotoxin antibodies improve survival. Pulmonary artery catheters have not been shown to improve outcome.

17.   Oxygen haemoglobin dissociation curve   **Answers: A C E**
The oxygen haemoglobin dissociation curve is sigmoid shaped and reaches a plateau at 70–100 mmHg (pO$_2$). A left shift is produced by a high pH, alkalosis, fall in pCO$_2$, fall in temperature and fall in 2,3 DPG. As a result of a left shift, less oxygen is released (a higher % saturation for a given pO$_2$, leading to a fall in oxygen delivery). Anaemia does not produce any shift of the curve but alters the % O$_2$ saturation of the blood.

18.   Angiotensin II   **Answers: D E**
Angiotensin II stimulates aldosterone synthesis and secretion through activity of a specific receptor found in the zona glomerulosa. It is one of the most potent endogenous vasoconstrictor agents and it inhibits renin release through a negative feedback loop. Renin stimulates the formation of angiotensin I from angiotensinogen. Angiotensin I is converted to angiotensin II in the lung.

19.   Baseline investigations   Answers: B C
Baseline investigations for a patient with major burns include routine haematology and biochemistry, carboxyhaemoglobin estimation, arterial blood gases, and CXR. Carbon monoxide has an increased affinity for haemoglobin, and displaces oxygen from the haemoglobin molecule, shifting the oxygen haemoglobin dissociation curve to the left. Glycosylated haemoglobin is used to assess recent blood glucose control in diabetics.

20.   Fluid replacement   Answers: A E
Excessive crystalloid administration results in increased filtration pressure, reduced colloid osmotic pressure, and increased capillary permeability. The end result is interstitial and intra-alveolar oedema, promoting the development of ARDS. Initial volume expansion is more quickly achieved with colloid rather than crystalloid. Neither colloid nor crystalloid administration prevents a fall in haematocrit level following blood loss. Stored blood has a low pH and infusion may exacerbate an existing acidosis. It is also high in potassium, and low in clotting factors and functioning platelets. Blood is the fluid of choice to replace ongoing haemorrhage and hypotension. Bleeding sites need to be urgently identified and controlled.

21.   Management of multi-traumatised patient   Answers: A B C
During the management of a multi-traumatised patient, primary and secondary surveys should be repeated frequently to ascertain deterioration in patient status. They guide any changes to treatment. Blood at the penile meatus, perineal bruising, or a high-riding prostate indicate urethral damage. They are thus contraindications to urethral catheterization, without a preceding urethrogram to assess urethral integrity. Cribriform plate fractures may lead to intra-cranial passage of a per-nasally inserted gastric tube. In such circumstances gastric tubes should be placed per orum. Skull X-rays are not usually valuable in making management decisions in the initial major trauma situations or in the absence of penetrating cranial injuries. They are time consuming, difficult to interpret, and may impair the resuscitation of the patient. Blood pressure itself is not a reliable measure of actual tissue perfusion.

22. Pelvic trauma
Answers: A B

To destabilise a ring structure mechanically, loss of fixation in two or more points is required. Acetabular fractures are usually evident on AP X-rays of the pelvis, though some posterior fracture-dislocations may not be obvious. Acetabular fractures are due to forceful impaction by the femoral head. Acetabular fractures are best visualised on CT scan. Post-traumatic arthritis is common.

23. Thoracic trauma
Answers: A C E

Traumatic rupture of the thoracic aorta usually follows rapid deceleration, and is usually fatal. The commonest site of injury is just distal to the origin of the left subclavian artery. Arch aortography is still the 'gold standard' and the diagnostic modality of choice.

24. Partial thickness burns
Answers: A C E

Partial thickness burns commonly result from contact with hot fluids. There is blistering, broken epidermis and swelling. These burns are characteristically red or mottled and have a weeping surface. They are painful and sensitive to air.

25. Tissue hypoxia
Answers: A C D

Pulmonary ventilation-perfusion mismatch results from contusions, haematomas and alveolar collapse. Reduced ventilation results in hypercarbia. Hypovolaemia from blood loss and changes in intra-thoracic pressure relationships (from tension or open pneumothoraces) clearly compromise oxygen exchange.

26. Glasgow Coma Scale
Answers: A E

GLASGOW COMA SCALE

Eye opening			Verbal response	
spontaneous	4		orientated	5
to speech	3		confused conversation	4
to pain	2		inappropriate words	3
none	1		incomprehensible sounds	2
			none	1

Motor response	
obeys commands	6
localises pain	5
normal flexion (withdrawal)	4
normal flexion (decorticate)	3
extension (decerebrate)	2
none (flaccid)	1

The Glasgow Coma Scale was designed as a method of following the evolvement of neurological disability and prognosticating future recovery. Eye opening is scored on a scale of 1–4, the best verbal response to stimulation on a scale of 1–5, and the best motor response to stimulation on a scale of 1–6. Therefore, the total score ranges from 3–15. Vital signs do not impact on the score. An unconscious patient with no eye opening, and no verbal or motor response to stimuli scores 3. A neurologically normal and alert patient scores 15. A deteriorating Glasgow Coma Scale is of great clinical significance and indicates progressive cerebral injury.

27.   Pulmonary thromboembolism   **Answers: A C D E**
Pulmonary thromboembolism may produce the classical ECG pattern of $S_1Q_3T_3$, and reduced arterial pCO_2 tension due to hyperventilation. Mismatched ventilation-perfusion defects on lung scan may be found. On CXR a pleural effusion, pulmonary atelectasis, area of oligaemia, and a raised hemidiaphragm may be observed. Obstruction to the pulmonary circulation on angiography (which provides the definitive diagnosis) may be observed.

28.   Swan-Ganz catheterisation   **Answers: A C E**
Pulmonary artery occlusion (or wedge) pressure can be directly measured by Swan-Ganz catheterisation. Cardiac index and left ventricular stroke work can also be derived from these measurements using the Fick principle. FiO_2 (concentration of inspired oxygen) and end tidal CO_2 (concentration of expired CO_2) cannot be measured by Swan-Ganz catheterisation.

29.   Cutaneous naevi   **Answer: C**
When melanocytes drop off the epidermis into the dermis they are known as naevus cells. If these cells clump at the dermis/epidermis junction, the lesion is known as a junctional naevus. If cells only clump in the dermis, the lesion is known as an intradermal naevus. If clumping occurs at both sites, the lesion is known as a compound naevus. None of the three varieties have a high malignant potential, though malignant change does occur. Halo naevi are confined to the dermis, and malignant transformation is very rare.

30. Rectal anastomosis   Answers: A D

It is now well recognised that lower colorectal anastomoses (especially those below the peritoneal reflection) have a higher leak rate compared with higher anastomoses. There is no convincing evidence that single or double layered anastomoses, or the type of suture material used, provides any functional advantage. Stapled and handsewn anastomoses have similar clinical leak rates. Radiological leak rates are greater than clinical leak rates for both stapled and handsewn anastomoses. Radiological leakage in the absence of clinical manifestations is rarely of clinical importance.

31. Viral hepatitis   Answers: A D

There is good evidence that chronic hepatitis B and hepatitis C infection increases the risk of developing hepatocellular carcinoma. The acute illness of hepatitis C virus is generally less severe than that of hepatitis A or hepatitis B viruses. Patients rarely become jaundiced and there is a lower level of enzyme rise.

32. Actinomycosis infection   Answers: A B D

Actinomycosis is very sensitive to penicillin (antibiotic of choice). However, infection is frequently found in association with other bacteria, and therefore it is advisable to treat the patient with metronidazole as well. Pus requires appropriate drainage or excisional surgery together with antibiotics.

33. *Clostridium difficile*   Answers: A E

Clostridium difficile infections have increased six fold in the past few years. The ability of *Clostridium difficile* to induce disease depends on the fact that the bacterium must be ingested into the colonic flora, and then become established. This usually occurs because the normal flora is disturbed. Disturbance of colonic flora is usually due to antibiotics but chemotherapy (anti-neoplastic) drugs can also cause *Cl. difficile* infections. Third generation cephalosporins (e.g. ceftazidime) are strongly associated with *Cl. difficile* infection. Diarrhoea usually starts within a few days but up to 1–2 months may elapse before symptoms occur.

34.   Enlarging pituitary gland   **Answers: B E**

Pituitary tumours compress the lower decussating fibres in the optic chiasm causing upper quadrantic bitemporal hemianopia. Pupillary reflexes become increasingly affected with progressive destruction of the optic axons (which mediate the afferent arc of the reflex). Cavernous sinus drainage occurs mainly through the inferior petrosal sinus and is therefore uncompromised. The sella turcica and anterior clinoid processes become eroded, but the more distant posterior clinoid processes, separated from the gland by the internal carotid arteries, ophthalmic arteries and cavernous sinus, are spared.

35.   Spinal cord hemi-transection   **Answers: All false**

The perception of noxious stimuli is lost contralaterally below the lesion. Ipsilateral motor signs below the lesion are those of an upper motor neurone lesion. The biceps reflex tests the C5/6 spinal segments; thus the reflex is intact and normal. Wasting of the muscles of the thenar eminence (recurrent muscular branch of the median nerve, often with double innervations from the ulnar nerve: C8/T1), claw hand (ulnar nerve: C7-T1), and winged scapula (long thoracic nerve: C5-7) are all signs of lower motor neurone lesions, below the upper level of the C7 spinal cord segment, and thus would not feature in this case.

36.   Thoracic duct   **Answers: A C E**

The thoracic duct ascends anterior to the posterior intercostal vessels and has several valves. At the thoracic inlet, it lies to the left of the oesophagus and arches forward over the dome of the left pleura. The right bronchomediastinal trunk drains into the right subclavian vein.

37.   Hilum of the left lung   **Answers: A B D E**

The phrenic nerve lies anterior, the vagus posterior, to the left hilum. The left main bronchus lies inferior to the pulmonary artery and does not divide before entering the lung. The hilum is separated from the aortic arch and descending thoracic aorta by the vagus nerve.

38.   Aortic arch   **Answers: B D E**

The apex of the arch, which gives attachment to the pretracheal fascia, lies posteroinferior to the left brachiocephalic vein. The lower border of the arch lies in the transthoracic plane and on the left is directly related to the left pulmonary artery (the superior vena cava lies over the right pulmonary artery). The arch is symmetrically covered by the pleura from both sides, which meet in the midline behind the manubriosternal joint.

39.   **Intervertebral disc collapse**   **Answer: E**

An L5-S1 disc presses on the S1 spinal nerve (the L5 nerve passes above the prolapsed disc in the intervertebral foramen and thus escapes damage). At the level of prolapse, the spinal canal contains the cauda equina and not cord *per se*. The S1 dermatome lies over the lateral malleolus. Exaggerated reflexes are diagnostic of an upper motor neurone lesion. The S2 dermatome occupies the posterior aspect of the calf.

40.   **Prolongation of APTT**   **Answers: B D E**

The activated partial thromboplastin time (APTT) measures the integrity of the intrinsic and common coagulation pathways and so is sensitive to a deficiency of factors VIII, IX, XI, XII and to a lesser extent factors V, X and prothrombin. The APTT is prolonged in patients on warfarin, except in the very early stages, due to impaired synthesis of the vitamin K dependent factors II, VII, IX and X. Intravenous heparin potentiates the activity of the endogenous anticoagulant anti-thrombin III and prolongs the APTT by inhibition of the intrinsic and common pathway factors. Low molecular heparin selectively inhibits factor Xa and at therapeutic doses has little or no effect on the APTT. Thromboprophylaxis with subcutaneous heparin does not usually prolong the APTT. Lupus anticoagulant is an example of a coagulation factor inhibitor which has affinity to factors in the intrinsic pathway. The presence of a lupus anticoagulant impairs the function of these factors and so prolongs the APTT.

41.   **Haemophilia**   **Answers: D E**

Haemophilia A is a sex-linked inherited disorder characterised by a complete or partial deficiency of factor VIII. Heterozygous female carriers have a Factor VIII level of approximately 50% although some individuals have sufficiently low levels to cause clinical symptoms. Severe disease (Factor VIII <1%) is characterised by painful joint and muscle bleeds which eventually lead to a chronic arthropathy. Rarer manifestations include pseudotumour formation following muscle bleeds, nerve entrapment, compartment syndromes, haematuria and post-traumatic intra-cranial bleeds. Significant mortality arises from replacement therapy associated with HIV, hepatitis B and hepatitis C infection. Haemophilia B is a sex-linked disorder arising from deficiency of factor IX. The clinical pattern is similar to haemophilia A.

ANSWERS – Core Paper 1

42.   Fresh frozen plasma   **Answers: B C D**

Fresh frozen plasma (FFP) contains all the non-cellular components of blood, including all clotting factors, immunoglobulin, albumin and other plasma proteins. Although FFP contains some fibrinogen, in situations such as severe hypofibrinogenaemia associated with disseminated intravascular coagulation, it is usual to supplement FFP with cryo-precipitate which has a higher fibrinogen concentration. FFP is supplied as 150–200 ml units separated from a single whole blood donation or in some centres, as a 300 ml unit obtained from a single donor plasmapheresis. Storage is at -30°C and may be for up to one year. FFP should be thawed in a waterbath in the transfusion laboratory and administered within four hours usually at a dose of 12–15 ml/kg. Repeated transfusion should subsequently be prescribed according to the results of a post-transfusion coagulation screen. Donor FFP may contain anti-A or anti-B antibodies which can sometimes cause dramatic haemolysis of recipient red cells. FFP is therefore usually issued as ABO compatible.

43.   Coagulation defects   **Answers: A D**

Fresh frozen plasma (FFP) is appropriate for the pre-operative correction of global clotting defects associated with liver disease or if urgent correction of warfarin anticoagulation is required. FFP should be restricted to patients with a PT > 18 s or APTT > 55 s. Cryoprecipitate may be added if the fibrinogen is < 1.0 g/l but should not be used alone. Specific factor concentrates are available for most single clotting factor deficiencies including haemophilia A. Because of the short half-life of many of the clotting factors in FFP, administration should be as close to surgery as possible. Intravenous vitamin K (0.5–1 mg) is a useful adjunct to FFP in the correction of warfarin associated bleeding. It may be used alone if bleeding is trivial or if surgery can be deferred for 24 hours

44.   Red cell units   **Answers: B D**

After viral screening, red cells are separated from whole blood and resuspended in an optimal additive solution, usually SAG-M (sodium chloride, adenine, glucose and mannitol). Each unit has a volume of 280 ml ± 60 and has a shelf life of 35 days when stored at 2–6 °C. All units are ABO and rhesus D phenotyped and when issued, must be ABO and rhesus D compatible but not necessarily identical to the donor. As a final precaution, red cells are crossmatched against recipient serum unless in a transfusion emergency. Once issued, red cells must be administered within five hours of leaving the transfusion laboratory. As red cells are stored, potassium and hydrogen ions leak into the suspension medium and this may cause biochemical disturbances in the recipient if large volumes are transfused.

45. Haemolytic transfusion reaction   **Answers: B D E**

Acute haemolytic transfusion reactions are the result of administration of ABO incompatible blood:- group A, B or AB to a group O recipient; group A or AB to a group B recipient; or group B or AB to a group A recipient. Clerical error outside the transfusion laboratory is the commonest cause. Clinically the reaction can be recognised by very rapid onset of agitation, flushing, pain at the venepuncture site, abdomen, flank or chest, a fever, hypotension, haemoglobinuria or haemoglobinaemia. This may be clinically indistinguishable from the effects of transfusing blood contaminated with Gram-negative organisms. Management should be the immediate cessation of transfusion, supportive measures and confirmation of the diagnosis with serological and haematological investigations.

46. Statistical analysis   **Answers: C E**

Finding results that are not statistically significant when the populations are different is known as Type II error. You miss the difference due to some combination of small sample size or high variability. Finding a statistically significant result when the populations are identical is called Type I error. You happen to randomly obtain larger values in one group and smaller values in the other, and the difference is large enough to generate a p-value < 0.05. The Gaussian (normal) distribution plays an important role in statistical analysis. An unpaired t-test compares two groups on the assumption that the two populations are Gaussian. Paired t-tests compare two paired groups. Parametric tests are used when data from population groups follow a Gaussian distribution. Non-parametric tests are used when data from the population group do not follow a Gaussian distribution.

47. Clinical audit   **Answers: B C E**

Clinical audit in surgical practice can be led by any interested appointed party (e.g. medical or nursing staff, or administrator) with access to the required data. Audit assesses some aspect or endpoint(s) associated with a particular clinical intervention, with a view to assessing outcomes or effects. It offers the ability to alter clinical practice if findings suggest improvements can be made (completing the audit cycle). Detailed clinical information is not always required if only a particular aspect of outcome or care is being assessed.

SECTION 2 – EMQs

Microbiology following skin trauma

61. Carbuncles	A	*Staphylococcus aureus*
62. Infected dog bites	C	*Pasteurella multocida*
63. Cellulitis	B	*Streptococcus pyogenes*
64. Styes	A	*Staphylococcus aureus*
65. Infected human bites	D	*Streptococcus milleri*
66. Infected leg ulcers	A	*Staphylococcus aureus*

Carbuncles and styes are primarily caused by *Staphylococcus aureus*. Infected leg ulcers usually have mixed flora but are mostly due to *Staphylococcus aureus*. Other organisms include coliforms, *Pseudomonas aeruginosa*, and anaerobes. *Pasteurella multocida* is frequently present in infected dog bites and cat scratches, though others may include many anaerobes. Infected human bites contain *Streptococcus milleri*, Haemophilus species, and other oral anaerobes. Cellulitis is most commonly caused by *Streptococcus pyogenes*, though other species such as Gram-negatives may be involved.

Wounds

67. The small bowel has been entered but without significant spillage of contents	C	Clean-contaminated
68. A non-infected biliary tract has been entered	C	Clean-contaminated
69. Crush wound to the leg	D	Contaminated
70. An infected genito-urinary tract has been entered	D	Contaminated
71. Scalpel incision for a ganglion excision	B	Clean
72. Inadvertent incision into the vagina	C	Clean-contaminated

Wounds can be divided into three categories:

Clean:	non-traumatic; respiratory, gastrointestinal and genito-urinary tracts not entered.
Clean-contaminated:	gastrointestinal, respiratory or genito-urinary tract entered without significant spillage
Contaminated:	traumatic wound; gross spillage from the gastrointestinal; entrance into the genito-urinary or biliary tract in the presence of infected urine or bile.

Burns in children

73.	Burns to all the head and neck	F	18%
74.	Burns to all the anterior trunk (chest and abdomen)	F	18%
75.	Burns to all the male genitalia	A	1%
76.	Burns to all the posterior trunk (upper and lower back)	F	18%
77.	Burns to the whole anterior aspect of one leg	C	7%
78.	Burns to the whole aspect of one arm	D	9%
79.	Burns to the posterior aspect of both legs	E	14%

The relative body surface areas in children are different to adults. The head and neck make up a larger proportion of total body area at 18% and the legs a smaller proportion at 14%. Other regions are the genitals (1%), the anterior trunk (chest and abdomen) (18%), the posterior trunk (upper and lower) (18%), and each arm (9%).

Hormone secreting tumours

80.	Testicular teratoma	E	α–fetoprotein
81.	Bronchial carcinoma	F	ACTH
82.	Medullary thyroid carcinoma	A	Calcitonin
83.	Carcinoid tumour	C	5 hydroxytryptamine
84.	Hypernephroma	B	Erythropoietin
85.	Pituitary adenoma	D	Growth hormone

α-fetoprotein is secreted in high amounts by hepatocellular carcinomas (90% cases) and teratomas. Bronchial carcinomas may secrete a variety of hormones including ACTH, Cortisol, ADH and parathormone. Medullary thyroid carcinoma is known to secrete calcitonin (from parafollicular C cells) and the latter is a good tumour marker.
Renal carcinoma may present with polycythaemia as part of a paraneoplastic syndrome. This is due to excess secretion of erythropoietin.

Paraneoplastic syndromes

86.	Myasthenia gravis	E	Thymoma
87.	Polycythaemia	D	Renal carcinoma
88.	Hypercalcaemia	A	Multiple myeloma
89.	Hyperglycaemia	B	Pancreatic carcinoma

Myasthenia gravis is seen with some thymic tumours. Polycythaemia may result from tumours of the kidney or cerebellum due to increased erythropoietin production. Hypercalcaemia results from bone mobilisation from bony metastases and ectopic parathormone. It is most commonly seen in myeloma, breast and lung cancer. Pancreatic carcinoma may lead to hyperglycaemia. Gout sometimes accompanies lymphoma. Thrombophlebitis migrans is especially associated with lung and pancreatic cancer.

Peripheral nerve anatomy

90.	Tongue insensitive to touch and taste	B	Lingual nerve
91.	Dry eye, blunted tastes, paralysis of buccinator	A	Facial nerve
92.	Left-sided ptosis and dilated pupil	F	Oculomotor nerve
93.	Left-sided ptosis and constricted pupil	H	Cervical sympathetic trunk
94.	Clouding vision left eye, intact corneal reflex, burning pain over forehead and left eye, no ptosis or diplopia	C	Ophthalmic nerve

- Mal-application of dental forceps during extraction of a lower 7 or 8 can crush or sever the lingual nerve as it passes in a groove in the alveolar bone under the gum. Such lesions cause ipsilateral loss of proprioception from the muscles of the tongue, predisposing to laceration between the occlusal surfaces of the teeth. The lingual nerve also subserves general sensation to the mucous membrane over the anterior two-thirds of the tongue (taste is from the chorda tympani nerve - VII).

- Facial paralysis is often not noticed by patients with Bell's palsy, but other ipsilateral symptoms including dry eye (loss of lacrimal secretion) leading to corneal ulceration, impaired vision, some loss of taste (from the anterior two-thirds of the tongue), inability to close the mouth, and the collection of food in the vestibule (paralysis of the buccinator muscle) are of concern. This particular lesion is located in the nerve at or before the origin of the superior petrosal branch.

- IIIrd nerve lesions give rise to ipsilateral ptosis (paralysis of the striated component of the levator palpebrae superioris muscle), and pupillary dilatation (paralysis of the constrictor pupillae muscle). There is also an ipsilateral depressed lateral (down and out) strabismus (paralysis of all extraocular muscles, except superior oblique and lateral rectus).

- In Horner's syndrome, signs include ptosis (paralysis of the smooth muscle component of the levator palpebrae superioris muscle), and pupillary constriction (paralysis of the dilator pupillae muscle).

- In herpes zoster infection of the ophthalmic division of V, a rash appears over the forehead from the vertex to the upper eye lid extending over the ala of the nose (the external nasal branch of the nasociliary nerve). If the cornea is involved (ciliary branch), blindness may result from scarring.

Structures in the transpyloric plane

95. Gives off a branch which ascends between the trachea and oesophagus
96. Gives attachment to pre-vertebral fascia
97. Has a vestigial ligamentous attachment
98. Has a compound articulation with a secondary cartilaginous joint
99. Crosses the midline
100. Has the carina located in the plane
101. Meet in the midline

102. Receives the azygos vein

G Vagus nerve
D T4 vertebra
F Left pulmonary artery
H 2nd costal cartilage
J Thoracic duct
A Trachea
C Mediastinal parietal pleura
B Superior vena cava

- The left recurrent laryngeal nerve is given off by the vagus as it descends between the concavity of the aortic arch and left pulmonary artery. The left recurrent laryngeal nerve loops round the ligamentum arteriosum and ascends into the neck in a groove between the trachea and oesophagus.
- The prevertebral fascia fuses with the T4 vertebra.
- The ligamentum arteriosum is a remnant of the fibrosed ductus arteriosus, which interconnects the left pulmonary artery with the concavity of the aortic arch in the foetus.
- The sternocostal joint has an intra-articular ligament (connecting the 2nd costal cartilage to the fibrocartilage of the manubriosternal joint) and two synovial cavities (an upper compartment for articulation with the manubrium, and a lower compartment for articulation with the body of the sternum).
- The thoracic duct gains the left side and continues its ascent on the bodies of the thoracic vertebrae.
- The trachea divides slightly to the right of the midline. The carina is a keel shaped cartilage at the bifurcation.
- The mediastinal pleura on each side meet in the midline in front of the aortic arch.
- The azygos vein arches over the hilum of the right lung, indenting the upper lobe before joining the superior vena cava.

Blood

103.	Inhibits platelet aggregation	C	Aspirin
104.	Prolongs prothrombin time	E	Warfarin
105.	Is an inhibitor of fibrinolysis	F	Aprotinin
106.	Is a major source of clotting factors	A	Fresh frozen plasma
107.	Fractionated forms are more efficacious	D	Heparin

Fresh frozen plasma contains all the clotting factors when first prepared but the concentration of some factors falls very rapidly. Streptokinase activates plasminogen to form plasmin which degrades fibrin thereby dissolving clot. Aspirin inhibits platelet aggregation. Heparin impedes the procoagulant interaction of thrombin with fibrinogen and promotes the anticoagulant action of antithrombin III. Factors II, VII, IX and X are synthesised by an enzyme which requires vitamin K as a cofactor. Synthesis of these factors is inhibited by warfarin and the extent of this effect is measured by the prolongation of the prothrombin time. Aprotinin is a proteolytic enzyme inhibitor and therefore has 'procoagulant' activity.

Inherited coagulation disorders

108.	PT 12 s, APTT 56 s, Plts 70	B	von Willebrand's disease
109.	PT 45 s, APTT 28 s, Plts 345	C	Factor VII deficiency
110.	PT 16 s, APTT 62 s, Plts 380	A	Haemophilia A
111.	PT 35 s, APTT 45 s, Plts 321	D	Factor X deficiency

For this question it is essential to understand that deficiencies of extrinsic factor pathway factors (VII) cause prolongation of the PT; deficiencies of intrinsic factors (XII, IX and VIII) cause prolongation of the APTT and deficiencies of common factors (II, V, X) cause prolongation of both PT and APTT. Haemophilia A (factor VIII deficiency) and von Willebrand's disease (in which factor VIII has a reduced half life) may be difficult to distinguish in the laboratory. Some varieties of von Willebrand's disease are however associated with thrombocytopenia. Glanzmann's disease is a rare inherited platelet function disorder. In common with acquired platelet function disorders such as in aspirin therapy, the platelet count and coagulation screen are normal.

Renal failure

112. Prolonged hypotension, oliguria   C Acute tubular necrosis
     with subsequent recovery of
     urinary function
113. 3l of iv fluids followed by 3 units H Pulmonary oedema
     of packed cells over four hours
114. Lacerated liver and perforated   F Prerenal renal failure
     duodenum. Urine output
     improved after iv fluids

A story of prolonged hypotension followed by a period of oliguria/anuria which eventually makes a complete recovery is typical of acute tubular necrosis (ATN). Cortical necrosis may produce a similar picture but does not usually recover.

Any patient who has received large volumes of fluid and becomes hypoxic must be considered to have pulmonary oedema until proven otherwise. It is particularly likely to occur in those with compromised cardiovascular or renal function, especially the elderly.

The lady with the liver laceration although oliguric initially, did not develop and progress to acute renal failure. Once renal perfusion was restored she was able to produce urine normally. This suggests that the cause of the renal impairment was poor perfusion, secondary to hypovolaemia. This is a pre-renal cause of renal failure and, if inadequately treated, will progress to acute tubular necrosis (see above), an intrinsic cause of renal failure.

Cerebral injury

115. Bleeding from nose, mouth and   E   Basal skull fracture
right ear, conscious
116. Sudden onset of severe occipital   B   Subarachnoid haemorrhage
headache
117. Fell over one week ago, now   A   Subdural haematoma
flucuating level of consciousness
118. Initial loss of consciousness for   D   Extradural haematoma
10 mins, normal for one hour
and subsequent drop in conscious
level

Basal skull fracture is suggested by a number of signs including bleeding or CSF leaking from the nose or ears. Battle's sign (bruising around the mastoid) and 'raccoon eyes' (periorbital ecchymoses) usually occur later. Subarachnoid haemorrhage is characterised by a sudden, dramatically severe onset of headache. Subdural haematomas often occur following the rupture of bridging veins in the elderly and are easy to miss because of the fluctuating levels of consciousness. A lucid phase is classical in an extradural haematoma. Treatment is usually emergency drainage.

Ventilation

119. Application of positive airway   B   CPAP
pressure throughout all phases of
ventilation
120. Used to improve oxygenation in   H   Reversed I:E ratio
respiratory failure in addition to
PEEP
121. Ventilation delivered through the   D   High frequency jet insufflation
cricothyroid membrane
122. Ventilation mode for fixed tidal   F   Volume controlled ventilation
volume
123. Best ventilation for poorly   E   Pressure controlled ventilation
compliant lungs
124. Used to reduce FiO_2 requirement   A   PEEP
and improve oxygenation
125. Pre-set minute volume, but   C   Intermittent mandatory
patient allowed to breathe   ventilation
spontaneously

In general, ventilators control either the volume or pressure of gas delivered to the patient. When ventilating a patient who has a low arterial pressure of oxygen, oxygenation can be improved by a combination of increasing the FiO_2, adding positive end expiratory pressure (PEEP), or by reversing the inspiratory: expiratory (I:E) ratio. The latter is most useful when the lungs are poorly compliant (stiff), but may be detrimental to CO_2 transfer. If the patient's major problem is hypercapnia, increasing the minute volume (by increasing rate and/or tidal volume) will lower the end tidal CO_2 (a reflection of alveolar and arterial CO_2).

Cardiovascular physiology

126. Passive left ventricular filling   C Throughout phase 5
127. Closure of the mitral valve   B Start of phase 2
128. Opening of the aortic valve   A End of phase 2
129. Second heart sound   F During phases 1 and 2
130. Left ventricular ejection   D Phase 1
131. The QRS complex   E Phase 3

Phase 1	Atrial contraction (atrial systole).
Phase 2	Isometric ventricular contraction lasts from the closure of the AV valves until ventricular pressure exceeds aortic and pulmonary pressures and the aortic and pulmonary valves open.
Phase 3	Ventricular ejection, lasts until the aortic and pulmonary valves close.
Phase 4	Isometric ventricular relaxation lasts until the AV valves open.
Phase 5	Passive ventricular filling

END OF CORE PAPER 1

1. Atrial natriuretic peptide **Answers: B C D**

Atrial natriuretic peptide (ANP) is a vasoactive compound, which increases renal blood flow within the kidney. ANP raises GFR, lowers renin production and causes natriuresis and diuresis. Water intake and salt appetite are both decreased. It has not been shown to be effective in the treatment of acute tubular necrosis.

2. Haemorrhage **Answers: B C E**

Haemorrhage is defined as acute loss of circulating blood. The normal adult blood volume is approximately 7% of body weight (therefore a 70 kg male has a 5 litre circulating blood volume), and in children is approximately 8–9% of body weight. The blood volume of obese patients is estimated by their ideal body weight, as their true weight gives an over-estimation of blood volume. Tachycardia is the earliest measurable sign of haemorrhage.

3. Diagnosis of ARDS **Answer: A**

ARDS is the most extreme manifestation of acute lung injury. Diagnostic criteria include:

- known cause of acute lung injury e.g. aspiration, massive transfusion
- diffuse alveolar shadows on chest X-ray (early radiographic signs are non-specific)
- absence of cardiac failure diagnosed by wedge pressure below 18 mmHg
- hypoxaemia defined as $FiO_2/PaCO_2 > 27$

The final common pathway involves neutrophil activation, inflammatory mediators and release of free radicals with increased alveolar capillary permeability. Various modes of ventilation are employed in the management (high frequency jet ventilation and extracorporeal membrane oxygenation) including prone position ventilation.

4. Acute inhalational injury **Answers: B C D**

Clinical indicators suggestive of acute inhalational injury include a history of confinement in a burning environment or history of explosion, facial burns, carbonaceous sputum, oesophageal carbon deposits, or singeing of the eyebrows, eye lashes or nasal hair.

5.   Total parenteral nutrition   Answers: B D

The essential components of total parenteral nutrition are nitrogen, carbohydrate, fat, minerals (calcium, magnesium, iron, zinc, manganese, copper, fluoride, iodine, chloride) and vitamins.

6.   Intra-operative heat loss   Answers: A B D

During anaesthesia, a patient inhales dry gases and exhales gas saturated with water vapour. Forming this water vapour consumes heat. A condenser-humidifier 'recycles' this water vapour reducing heat loss. Low flow anaesthesia recycles water vapour in a similar fashion. By contrast, volatile (i.e. evaporating) surgical sterilising agents may cause substantial heat loss as may the evaporation of water from bowel exposed to a dry theatre atmosphere. A 'bowel bag' reduces evaporation from exposed viscera. A laminar flow theatre blows air over the patient increasing heat loss by evaporation and convection.

7.   Diabetic emergencies   Answer: All false

Patients with Type I diabetes do not make their own insulin and require an exogenous supply. If they do not receive insulin they metabolise their carbohydrate and lipid reserve resulting in a high blood glucose and ketones (diabetic ketoacidosis). Initial treatment is with insulin not glucose. If a Type I diabetic receives too much insulin he/she may become hypoglycaemic. Type II diabetics make sufficient insulin to control their lipid metabolism but inadequate amounts to reduce their blood glucose into the normal range. Type II diabetics, therefore, usually suffer hypERglycaemia NOT hypOglycaemia or ketoacidosis.

Diabetic coma may result from hypOglycaemia (Type I) or hypERglycaemic hyperosmolality (in non-ketotic coma in Type II patients). Glucose administration is essential in the former and does not exacerbate the latter.

8.   Shock   Answers: C E

Shock is the inadequate perfusion and delivery of tissues with oxygen and other nutrients. Of all the shock states, cardiogenic shock is unique in that cardiac output is reduced and the systemic arteriolar vessels constrict, increasing the SVR in an attempt to maintain the blood pressure. In all other shock states there is primary vasodilatation of inappropriate vascular beds causing maldistribution of blood flow to areas where it is not required. This inappropriate vasodilation causes a fall in SVR and blood pressure. Cardiac output increases passively as a result of reduced afterload on the heart and actively as a result of increased sympathetic drive. Cardiac index relates cardiac output to body surface area.

9. **Post-operative complications** Answers: B C E

Hyponatraemia after surgery is usually due to inappropriate fluid therapy with hypotonic intravenous fluids (e.g. 5% dextrose) and increased secretion of ADH (leads to water retention). Patients who have had upper abdominal incisions are more prone to developing respiratory complications as a result of increased pain. The most common respiratory complication following general anaesthesia is atelectasis. This usually presents with pyrexia and tachypnoea. It should be treated with physiotherapy and oxygen. Septic shock usually produces a clinical picture of warm dilated peripheries but in advanced states may cause peripheral vasoconstriction – cold, clammy extremities.

10. **Human albumin solution** Answers: A C E

Human albumin solution is a purified derivative of pooled whole blood donations and is subject to virus heat inactivation. 20 g units are supplied as a freeze dried product that is stable at room temperature either as 400 ml of 5% solution or 100 ml of 20% solution. The 20% solution is hyperosmolar and may expand the plasma volume by more than the volume infused. The most common clinical uses are in the treatment of hypoproteinaemic oedema in nephrotic syndrome and ascites in chronic liver disease. Human albumin solutions should not be used as acute volume replacement because there is no evidence that they offer advantages over alternative fluids. The 5% solution has a sodium content of 130–150 mmol/l and may precipitate hypernatraemia in susceptible individuals.

11. **Contraindications to non-small cell lung resection** Answers: A B C

The other major contraindications include vocal cord and phrenic nerve paralysis, tumour within 2 cm of the carina, cardiac tamponade, involvement of the main pulmonary artery, metastasis to the supra-clavicular lymph nodes and severe pulmonary hypertension. A patient with an $FEV_1 > 2.5$ l would be able to tolerate a pneumonectomy.

12. **Abdominal pain in HIV patients** Answers: A B E

Numerous organisms produce infection and abdominal pain in HIV-infected individuals. The well documented organisms include: cryptosporidium, cytomegalovirus, *Mycobacterium tuberculosis*, Salmonella, Shigella, Campylobacter, *Neisseria gonorrhoea*, *Treponema pallidum*, *Mycobacterium avium-intracellulare*, *Listeria monocytogenes*, *Entamoeba histolytica*, *Giardia lamblia*, *Isospora belli*, *Candida albicans*, Histoplasma, and Herpes simplex virus. Kaposi's sarcoma is a vascular tumour.

13. Hydatid disease   **Answers: B D**

Hydatid disease is caused by the tapeworm *Echinococcus granulosus*. The intermediate host is the sheep. Dogs become infested by eating sheep offal and subsequently pass tapeworm eggs in their stool, which in turn contaminate their fur. This leads to accidental human ingestion. Therefore, man acts as accidental intermediate hosts. Emergent embryos pass through the intestinal wall into the portal system and liver, and to other organs, where they develop into hydatid cysts. Hepatic lesions are often asymptomatic and discovered by chance on investigation of other problems. Diagnosis should be made on serological testing or typical appearances of cyst septation and daughter cysts on CT. Needle biopsy is associated with the risk of anaphylaxis and dissemination of infection.

14. Osteomyelitis   **Answers: C D E**

Haematogenous infection from a primary focus elsewhere in the body is the commonest cause of osteomyelitis in neonates and children. Although this mode of infection can occur in adults, the commonest cause in this age group is following a compound fracture. Staphylococcus is the commonest organism in all age groups. In children, streptococci and Gram-negatives are found less commonly. In adults a variety of organisms may be found but staphylococci predominate.

The treatment of osteomyelitis consists of analgesia, antibiotics and rest. If this fails, the abscess is drained through drill holes and the limb rested in a splint or plaster cast for several weeks.

15. *Clostridium difficile*   **Answers: C E**

Clostridium difficile infection is usually detected by identification of cytotoxin. Gram staining of faeces to detect the organism is unhelpful because it cannot distinguish it from many of the other organisms. The first step in treatment should be cessation of the precipitating antibiotic(s). The two principal therapies are oral vancomycin 125 mg tds for 7–10 days and oral metronidazole 400 mg tds for 7–10 days. There is some evidence that oral vancomycin may be more clinically effective than metronidazole. Complications of *Cl. difficile* infection include electrolyte disturbances, paralytic ileus and if pan-colitis develops – toxic megacolon, perforation and endotoxic shock.

16.   Sterilisation of surgical equipment   Answers: All true

The constituents of surgical equipment vary and hence different instruments will require different sterilisation techniques. Plastics and rubber can tolerate moisture, but may melt or be deformed by the extremes of heat, as with steam sterilisation or autoclaving. They are best sterilised by gas (ethylene oxide) sterilisation or chemical sterilisation, such as 2% aqueous glutaraldehyde, where heat doesn't play a significant role. Gas sterilisation is also used for delicate instruments that may otherwise corrode using the chemical technique.

Dry heat sterilisation is appropriate for equipment that can tolerate heat, but not moisture, or those that are not well penetrated by steam. Steam autoclaving is quick and effective, particularly for metal instruments and is commonly used to re-sterilise contaminated instruments if required quickly during a surgical procedure.

17.   Incisional biopsy   Answers: A C

Tissue from the centre of malignant lesions is often necrotic and will frequently provide insufficient information to establish a definitive diagnosis. Invasion may be multifocal and a single biopsy may not be representative of the whole of the lesion and therefore is insufficient to exclude a malignant process. Tissue should be taken from the junction of abnormal and normal tissue, as this gives the best chance of characterising the underlying histological abnormality. To prevent autolysis of tissue, specimens should be stored in formalin if there is going to be a delay with histological processing.

18.   Primary survey   Answers: A B E

According to ATLS teaching, primary survey includes:

A   Airway maintenance with cervical spine control
B   Breathing and ventilation
C   Circulation and haemorrhage control
D   Disability: neurological status
E   Exposure/environmental control - prevent hypothermia

The purpose of the primary survey is to identify and manage life-threatening injuries.

Abdominal, musculo-skeletal, and detailed neurological assessment form part of the secondary survey.

19.   Secondary survey   **Answers: A B C E**

The secondary survey is a head to toe assessment. It includes assessment of vital signs, all body systems (head, neck, chest, abdomen, extremities, neurological) and GCS scoring. Special procedures required for assessment such as diagnostic peritoneal lavage (DPL), X-rays, and laboratory studies are also conducted in this phase.

20.   Pelvic trauma   **Answers: C E F**

Injuries to the urethra, bladder, lumbosacral nerve roots, genitalia, rectum and pelvic contents often accompany pelvic fractures. About 90% of bleeding from pelvic trauma is from the fracture site or pelvic veins. Major bleeding is rarely arterial in origin. The prevailing philosophy is to tamponade the low pressure retroperitoneal bleeding by splinting the pelvis and transfusing. If this fails, pelvic vascular embolization is advocated. Open surgical approaches for haemostasis are associated with a high mortality. The overall mortality of open pelvic fractures approaches 50%, and reflects associated abdominal, rectal, thoracic and head injuries. Cystography requires at least two views to exclude a bladder rupture.

21.   Diaphragmatic rupture   **Answers: B C D**

Acute traumatic diaphragmatic rupture is more common on the left side, reflecting the degree of protection offered to the right diaphragm by the liver. Abdominal viscera (including spleen, stomach, omentum, and small bowel) frequently migrate into the chest, especially on the left side, causing cardiac and respiratory embarrassment. Once in the chest, migrated viscera are at risk of obstruction or strangulation. Visceral migration may result in cardiac and mediastinal displacement. Treatment is surgical and involves reduction and repair of abdominal viscera, closure of the diaphragmatic defect, and drainage of the pleural cavity.

22.   Gunshot wounds   **Answers: B D**

High velocity bullets have enormous kinetic energy and produce cavitational effects which can result in tissue necrosis distant from the bullet track. Gunshot wounds to the abdomen are associated with significant visceral injury in about 95% of cases, and laparotomy is mandatory. If an exit wound is absent, AXRs may help determine missile trajectory by tracing sites of entry to residual bullet fragments. Gunshot wounds are contaminated and broad spectrum antibiotics should be routinely administered.

23.   Burns   Answers: C D

Burns accelerate cellular metabolism and inactivate thermo-labile enzymes. They cause vascular injury which results in tissue ischaemia, and denaturing of protein.

24.   Skin grafts   Answers: A D

Full thickness grafts contain the entire thickness of papillary and reticular dermis, in addition to epidermis. Hence, they have higher metabolic demands than the thinner split skin grafts, because of this they require optimal conditions to 'take'. Full thickness grafts give superior quality, contour, colour match, durability and lack of wound contraction compared with split skin grafts. Post-auricular and eyelid skin are useful for full thickness grafts, as are the groin and flank.

25.   Femoral nerve injury   Answers: A D

The femoral nerve supplies the quadratus femoris muscle, the contracting fibres of which elicit the knee jerk. The nerve supplies the L2–4 dermatomes over the anterior skin of the thigh. The genito-femoral nerve mediates the cremasteric reflex. The saphenous nerve (L4), a branch of the femoral, innervates the skin over the medial malleolus. The lateral cutaneous nerve of the thigh, and the genito-femoral nerve, both branches of the lumbar plexus, also supply the L2 dermatome.

26.   Anaphylactic shock   Answers: A B

The mainstay of management of severe anaphylactic shock includes airway maintenance and oxygen, iv fluids, and subcutaneous adrenaline. Nebulised bronchodilators counteract bronchospasm. Other drugs which might be helpful include aminophylline and hydrocortisone. β–blockers are contraindicated as they lower blood pressure and may cause bronchoconstriction.

27.   Familial Adenomatous Polyposis   Answers: B D E

FAP is inherited as an autosomal dominant disease, with an incidence of 1 in 6,000–23,000 live births. There is an associated long arm deletion at q21–q22 of chromosome 5. About a third of cases are sporadic, arising as new mutations without a positive family history.

28.   Mastectomy   Answers: B D

Relative indications for mastectomy rather than conservative breast excision for breast cancer include multifocal disease, larger tumours, extensive DCIS, smaller breasts, salvage surgery, and patient choice. Axillary lymph node involvement is not an indication in its own right.

29. Malignant melanoma   **Answer: B**
Elective regional lymph node dissection (i.e. removal of clinically
uninvolved nodes draining the area of the primary) has not been shown
to increase survival of patients with cutaneous malignant melanoma.
Therapeutic regional lymph node excision (i.e. removal of clinically
involved nodes), however, does improve survival in a proportion of
patients, and is recommended in the absence of distant spread.
Melanoma is a relatively chemo-resistant and radio-resistant tumour.
Excision of solitary metastases, such as in the lung, is associated with
long-term survival in only a minority of patients.

30. Colorectal cancer   **Answers: B C D**
Testing for faecal occult blood has been shown to increase detection of
colorectal tumours confined to the bowel wall. The optimal period
between repeat testing has yet to be established. The haemoccult FOBT
relies on a peroxidase-type reaction, which turns a guaiac slide blue.

31. Paget's disease   **Answer: C**
Paget's disease of the nipple usually presents as a unilateral nipple
excoriation or scaling. Any persisting eczematous lesion of the nipple
requires biopsy for histological diagnosis. Paget's disease is associated
with an underlying ductal breast carcinoma in about 90% of cases,
which must be sought and treated. These associated breast carcinomas
have a better overall prognosis than breast cancer in the general
population.

32. Injury to radial nerve   **Answers: D E**
Abduction of the thumb is weakened, but not lost, after paralysis of the
abductor pollicis longus muscle (radial nerve), because the abductor
pollicis brevis muscle remains functional (median nerve). Extension of
the forearm is unaffected, since branches to the triceps muscle leave the
radial nerve before it enters the spiral groove. Despite paralysis of the
supinator muscle, supination is unaffected because the biceps muscle
remains functional (musculocutaneous nerve). Loss of sensation over the
first dorsal web and the brachioradialis tendon reflex (mainly C6 through
a branch coming off the radial nerve after leaving the spiral groove) are
features of radial nerve damage at this site.

33.   Ulnar nerve damage   Answers: B D

Ulnar nerve damage results in sensory loss over the hypothenar eminence, the whole of the little finger and the medial side of the ring finger. There is denervation of the flexor carpi ulnaris muscle, the ulnar half of the flexor digitorum profundus muscle, the muscles of the hypothenar eminence, the two ulnar lumbricals, all the interosseous muscles and the adductor pollicis muscle. Thus, both flexion of the little finger and abduction of the fingers are lost. Adduction of the wrist is still possible through the action of the extensor carpi ulnaris muscle. Claw hand, a feature of ulnar nerve damage at the wrist, is usually not present with high lesions at the elbow or above, because the distal interphalangeal joints cannot be flexed if the ulnar half of the flexor digitorum profundus muscle is paralysed.

34.   Subclavian arteries   Answers: All true

The thyroid gland is supplied by the inferior thyroid artery, a branch of the thyrocervical trunk. The internal thoracic artery supplies: (1) the breast, through anterior intercostal vessels, usually in the 2nd and 3rd intercostal spaces, (2) the rectus abdominis muscle, through the superior epigastric branch, and (3) the diaphragm, through the musculophrenic artery. The vertebral arteries supply the brain stem through the posterior inferior cerebellar arteries.

35.   Sympathetic chain   Answers: A B D

The thoracic sympathetic chain lies on the heads of the ribs, anterior to the posterior intercostal vessels, immediately under cover of the pleura, with the splanchnic nerves passing from the chain medially and anteriorly over the vertebral bodies. The thoracic sympathetic chain receives white rami from all intercostal nerves, and passes into the abdomen under the medial arcuate ligament of the diaphragm.

36.   Right coronary artery   Answers: All true

The SA node artery passes backwards between the right auricle and aorta, and forms a vascular ring around the termination of the superior vena cava. Arteriolar anastomoses between the terminations of the right and left coronary arteries exist, but are too few and small in calibre to compensate significantly in acute coronary artery occlusion.

37.   The trachea   Answers: A B E

The trachea is palpable in the jugular notch, bifurcates in the transthoracic plane and is innervated by the recurrent laryngeal nerves. The left main bronchus bifurcates inside the left lung and is not as vertical as the right main bronchus.

138

38.   Splenectomy   **Answers: B D**

Following splenectomy there is an early thrombocytosis, usually peaking between 7–10 days. There are increased circulating Howell-Jolly bodies (DNA fragments of nuclear origin, normally present in < 2% of circulating RBCs) and an increased proportion of target cells, sideroblasts (RBCs containing granules of free iron), and RBCs containing Heinz bodies (degraded haemoglobin, usually found in ageing RBCs). An early leucocytosis (usually neutrophils) is seen within hours and may last for several weeks. There is also increased platelet adhesiveness and platelet dysfunction.

39.   Microcytic anaemia   **Answers: A B D**

Microcytic anaemia is characteristic of iron deficiency and is usually associated with chronic bleeding from the gut or with menorrhagia. Microcytic anaemia may occur in α- or β-thalassaemia and in sideroblastic anaemia (defect in haem synthesis). Hereditary haemo-chromatosis is a disorder of iron absorption characterised by iron overload and has no direct haematological manifestations. The anaemia of chronic renal failure is normocytic.

40.   Anaemia   **Answers: A C D**

A normocytic normochromic anaemia is usually associated with chronic sepsis, inflammatory disorders and malignancy. It is often referred to as the 'anaemia of chronic disorders'. A normocytic anaemia may also occur in chronic, but not acute, renal failure due to a fall in erythropoietin production. A normal mean cell volume may result from a combined microcytic and macrocytic anaemia. This may be encountered in a combined iron and B_{12} or folate deficiency resulting from malabsorption typically after gastrectomy or in coeliac disease. In these cases, the diagnosis is usually obvious from a characteristically 'dimorphic' blood film.

41.   Bleeding disorders   Answers: A B

Bleeding time is a global test of small vessel haemostasis. It may be altered in thrombocytopenia, disorders of platelet function and collagen disorders affecting the vessel wall. However, the correlation with surgical bleeding is poor. Aspirin irreversibly inactivates platelets by inhibiting cyclo-oxygenase and therefore prolongs the bleeding time. Fibrinogen is manufactured in the liver and the synthesis is increased as part of the acute phase response. Reduced fibrinogen concentration may indicate a consumptive coagulopathy. The thrombin time (TT) is a measure of the conversion of fibrinogen to fibrin and is therefore prolonged in hypofibrinogenaemia. Inhibitors of fibrin polymerisation such as heparin, fibrin degradation products and severe hypo-albuminaemia also prolong the TT. Heparin may cause significant prolongation of the TT at concentrations well below that needed to prolong the APTT.

42.   von Willebrand's disease   Answers: B D E

von Willebrand's disease is the commonest inherited bleeding disorder in Caucasian populations and is usually autosomal dominant in inheritance. Affected individuals have reduced or dysfunctional von Willebrand factor (vWF), a protein normally present in platelets and endothelium. vWF stabilises Factor VIII in the circulation and mediates platelet adhesion at the site of vascular injury. The associated laboratory abnormalities therefore include a prolonged APTT (due to reduced Factor VIII), normal PT and a prolonged bleeding time (platelet adhesion defect). Clinically, affected individuals usually show a mild bleeding tendency with epistaxis, easy bruising, menorrhagia and gingival bleeding. Although factor VIII levels are characteristically reduced, levels are rarely sufficiently low to cause haemarthroses, the hallmark of haemophilia A. Pre-operative management usually involves treatment with desmopressin (which liberates platelet stores of vWF) or factor replacement with either intermediate purity factor VIII or a specific vWF concentrate.

43.   Platelets for transfusion   Answers: A C

Most blood transfusion centres supply platelets pooled from 4-6 individual donations suspended in plasma and supplied in volumes of approximately 200 ml. Platelets must be dispensed within five days. Immune mediated transfusion reactions are common but usually consist of mild febrile reactions caused by a recipient antibody response to donor plasma proteins or platelet antigens. Since all platelet preparations are contaminated with small quantities of red cells, they should preferably be ABO and rhesus D compatible with the recipient. Crossmatching of platelets is not required. Rhesus D negative women of child bearing age and younger must receive rhesus D negative platelets to avoid alloimmunisation and prevent rhesus haemolytic disease of the newborn.

44.   Blood transfusions   **Answers: All true**

Graft versus host disease (GVHD) is a near universally fatal condition caused by T-lymphocytes in donor blood and is characterised by fever, skin rash and gastrointestinal and liver dysfunction starting 4-30 days after transfusion. GVHD is prevented by using gamma-irradiated blood products. Lymphocyte contaminants in red cell products have immunosuppressant activity even in immunocompetent recipients. There is some evidence that recurrence of malignancy and sepsis is more common in heavily transfused patients undergoing surgery for malignant disease. Iron overload is inevitable in patients on long-term transfusion programmes. This may manifest as hepatic cirrhosis, endocrine insufficiency and cardiomyopathy. Post-transfusion purpura is a potentially fatal disorder that is due to the production of antibodies against foreign platelet antibodies after transfusion. Thrombocytopenia in the recipient occurs when these antibodies cross-react with the recipients own platelets. In the United Kingdom, blood products are not screened for the human T-cell leukaemia viruses (HTLV I and II) and a small number of patients acquire the lifelong risk of T-cell leukaemia from transfusion each year.

45.   Autologous transfusion   **Answers: A C**

Autologous pre-donation of blood for elective surgery prevents immuno-suppression and allergic reactions. Donation criteria consists of a haemoglobin of greater than 11 g/dl and elective procedures where blood loss is expected, for example, cardiac surgical operations (coronary artery bypass grafting, valve replacement). Active infection is a contraindication and donation is not advised if severe cardio-respiratory disease is present, for example, unstable angina or myocardial infarction within the last six months.

46.   Statistical analysis   **Answers: C E**

The mean of a set of values is the same as the average. The median is the middle value of the set of values. Standard deviation is a measure of the variability of a set of values: 68% of values lie within one SD on each side of the mean, and 95% within 2 SDs of the mean. Parametric tests are used for the assessment of data that follow a Gaussian distribution, and non-parametric tests for data not following a Gaussian (normal) distribution. The outcome of a rank or score has a limited range, and an arbitrary and artificial difference between scores. Such data cannot be Gaussian in distribution.

SECTION 2 – EMQs

Suture material

61.	Polyglactic acid (Vicryl)	A	Absorbable, braided, synthetic
62.	Nylon	D	Nonabsorbable, monofilament, synthetic
63.	Polyglyconate (Maxon)	B	Absorbable, monofilament, synthetic
64.	Polypropylene (Prolene)	D	Nonabsorbable, monofilament, synthetic
65.	Polydioxanone (PDS)	B	Absorbable, monofilament, synthetic
66.	Polyglycolic acid (Dexon)	A	Absorbable, braided, synthetic
67.	Silk	C	Nonabsorbable, braided, natural material

The common absorbable braided sutures include Vicryl and Dexon.
The common absorbable monofilament sutures include PDS, Maxon and Monocryl.
The common non-absorbable monofilament sutures include Prolene, Nylon and Steel wire.

Chemotherapy agents

68.	Cyclophosphamide	B	Alkylating agents
69.	Methylprednisolone	C	Corticosteroids
70.	Azathioprine	A	Anti-metabolites
71.	Cyclosporin	D	Anti-cytotoxic
72.	6-mercaptopurine	A	Anti-metabolites

Cyclophosphamide is activated by hepatic microsomal enzymes to produce several alkylating metabolites which cause cross-linking between DNA strands, preventing division of immunocompetent cells. Azathioprine is an anti-metabolite. It is metabolised to 6-mercaptopurine, within the liver, which is a purine antagonist reducing DNA and RNA synthesis in dividing cells. Cyclosporin acts at an intracellular level to block the proliferation of cytotoxic T-lymphocytes. Actions of corticosteroids include reduction of macrophage activity and motility, reduction of circulating T-cell populations, and stabilisation of lysosomal and cellular membranes.

Cancer therapy options

73.	Recurrent non-Hodgkin's lymphoma	C	Systemic chemotherapy
74.	Isolated pulmonary metastasis from colorectal cancer	D	Surgical resection
75.	Residual anal squamous cell carcinoma (SCC) after local radiotherapy	D	Surgical resection
76.	Metastatic prostatic carcinoma not involving bone	B	Hormonal manipulation
77.	Diffuse intracranial metastatic melanoma	A	Radiotherapy with steroids

Diffuse intracranial metastatic melanoma has an extremely poor prognosis. Short-term benefit may be achieved by radiotherapy with steroids, chemotherapy is of no benefit. Prolonged remission or even cure can be achieved using systemic chemotherapy for recurrent non-Hodgkin's lymphoma. Isolated pulmonary metastasis from colorectal cancer can be surgically removed with curative intent if the patient will tolerate a thoracotomy. Residual anal SCC after local radiotherapy is best treated by abdominoperineal resection with curative intent. Metastatic prostatic carcinoma not involving bone is best treated by hormonal manipulation; if bone is involved, radiotherapy is the treatment of choice, with or without internal fixation.

Mediastinal masses

78.	Thymic lesions	B	Anterior mediastinum
79.	Neural tumours	D	Posterior mediastinum
80.	Thyroid mass	A	Superior mediastinum
81.	Lymphoma	B	Anterior mediastinum
82.	Bronchogenic cyst	C	Middle mediastinum

The locations of mediastinal masses include:
Superior mediastinum: thyroid masses, lymph node enlargement, oesophageal tumours, aortic aneurysms, and parathyroid lesions.
Anterior mediastinum: thymic lesions, lymphoma, germ cell tumours, pleuropericardial cysts, lymph node enlargement.
Middle mediastinum: lymph node enlargement, bronchogenic cysts, enterogenic cysts.
Posterior mediastinum: neural tumours, thoracic meningocoele, oesophageal tumours, aortic aneurysms, paragangliomas.

Malignant melanoma

83. Occurs within a Hutchinson's melanotic freckle   C   Lentigo maligna melanoma

84. Has a predilection for sites of thick epidermis such as the sole of the foot   B   Acral lentiginous melanoma

85. Usually occurs on the face of elderly patients   C   Lentigo maligna melanoma

86. Is the commonest type of cutaneous malignant melanoma   A   Superficial spreading melanoma

Superficial spreading melanoma (65% of cases) is the commonest form of cutaneous malignant melanoma. Lentigo maligna is preceded by or occurs within a Hutchinson's melanotic freckle and is most commonly found on the face. Both of the above melanomas have a pronounced horizontal growth phase. Lentigo maligna melanoma and thin superficial spreading melanomas (<0.76 mm) have a good prognosis. Acral lentiginous melanomas have a predilection for sites of thick epidermis such as the sole of the foot, and have a poorer prognosis. Nodular melanomas have a pronounced vertical growth phase and hence a poor prognosis.

52. Resuscitation   Answers:

87. Pulse in a term neonate   F   Pulse 158/min

88. Blood pressure in a 2-year-old   B   Blood pressure 100/65 mmHg

89. Pulse in a 7-year-old   E   Pulse 100/min

90. Blood pressure in a term neonate   A   Blood pressure 70/40 mmHg

91. Respiratory rate in a 4-year-old   J   Respiratory rate 26/min

92. Respiratory rate in a 12-year-old   H   Respiratory rate 13/min

Age (years)	Pulse (/min)	Blood pressure (mmHg) systolic	Respirations (/min)
<1	110–160	70–90	30–40
1–4	95–140	80–100	25–30
5–11	80–120	90–110	20–25
≥ 12	60–100	100–120	12–20

It is important to be aware that children have different physiological normal ranges, otherwise the values may be misinterpreted.

Anatomy of cerebral vasculature

93. E   Vertebral artery
94. B   Posterior inferior cerebellar artery
95. A   Posterior cerebral artery
96. G   Striate arteries

- The medial medullary syndrome results from an infarct in the ventro-medial medulla oblongata after occlusion of the medullary branch of the vertebral artery. This results in destruction of the pyramid (contralateral hemiparesis), medial lemniscus (contralateral loss of all posterior column sensations) and rootlet of XII (ipsilateral lower motor neurone). With such alternating hemiplegias, the ipsilateral lower motor neurone component is the localising element.
- The lateral medullary syndrome results from an infarct in the lateral medulla oblongata after occlusion of the medullary branches of the posterior inferior cerebellar artery. There is destruction of the lateral spinothalamic tract (spinal lemniscus – contralateral loss of pain and temperature), nucleus ambiguus (paralysis of the muscles of the soft palate, pharynx, and larynx – difficulty in speaking and swallowing), and spinal tract and nucleus of V (ipsilateral loss of pain and temperature of the distribution of V).
- The posterior cerebral artery supplies the visual cortex. Occlusion of the artery thus causes the above signs and symptoms. Macular sparing is attributed to a dual blood supply to the occipital pole from both the posterior and middle cerebral arteries.
- Striate artery occlusion is the commonest cause of a stroke, affecting the posterior limb of the internal capsule, where both the descending corticospinal/corticobulbar projections, the ascending spinothalamic and the trigeminal sensory tracts to the thalamus are located.

ANSWERS – Core Paper 2

Anatomy of the heart

97.	Location of the sinoatrial node	I	Sulcus terminalis
98.	Originates from the anterior aortic sinus	A	Right coronary artery
99.	Overlies the left coronary artery	J	Left atrial appendage
100.	Drains into the right atrium	B	Coronary sinus
101.	Is connected to the largest papillary muscle	F	Anterior cusp of the mitral valve
102.	Lies posterior to the left atrium	K	Oblique pericardial sinus
103.	Location of the bundle of His	C	Membranous interventricular septum
104.	Location of the atrioventricular node	H	Interatrial septum

- The sinoatrial node lies over the sulcus terminalis of the right atrium.
- The right coronary artery originates from the anterior aortic sinus; the left from the left posterior sinus.
- Both atrial appendages overlie their respective coronary arteries.
- The coronary sinus drains into the right atrium just above the septal cusp of the tricuspid valve.
- The anterior cusp of the mitral valve is large, with a massive papillary muscle giving rise to multiple chordae tendinae attached along the edge of the cusp. The muscle prevents herniation of the cusp into the left atrium during systole when the cusp has to withstand the pressure of blood flowing over it towards the aortic opening.
- The oblique sinus separates the left atrium from the oesophagus posteriorly.
- The atrioventicular bundle of His traverses the membranous part of the interventricular septum before dividing into left and right bundle branches which travel towards the ventricular apices in the muscular interventricular septum.
- The atrioventricular node lies in the interatrial septum to the left of the opening of the coronary sinus.

Interpretation of the full blood count

105.Hb 21.3, WBC 14 (N 10, L 4), Plt 490	E	Polycythaemia rubra vera
106.Hb 12.2, WBC 298 (N 2, L 296), Plt 160	B	Chronic lymphocytic leukaemia
107.Hb 14.5, WBC 5.4 (N 3.8, L 1.3), Plt 25	C	Idiopathic thrombocytopenic purpura (ITP)
108.Hb 9.8, WBC 1.1 (N 0.5, L 0.6), Plt 45	A	Myelofibrosis
109.Hb 13.5, WBC 98 (N 82, L 16), Plt 640	D	Leukaemoid reaction

Isolated thrombocytopenia as in stem 3 is easy to attribute to idiopathic thrombo-cytopenic purpura. The severe pancytopenia (stem 4) is best explained by myelofibrosis in which fibrotic changes in the marrow lead to impairment of the production of all three cell lineages. Polycythaemia rubra vera is the only possibility for an elevated Hb but note that this is often accompanied by high white cell and platelet count. A very high white cell count can be narrowed down by the differential. If the cells are lymphoid, the likely diagnosis is chronic lymphocytic leukaemia or possibly acute leukaemia in which case there is usually a background pancytopenia. Very high neutrophil counts may represent chronic myeloid leukaemia but more frequently represent a leukaemoid reaction in response to sepsis. The platelet count may be raised in both of these examples.

Anticoagulant treatment regimens

110. D Tinzaparin 3500 u/kg *od.*
111. E Tinzaparin 175 u/kg *od.*
112. C Unfractionated heparin intravenously to maintain an APTT ratio of 2.5–3.5

Heparin is used in the prophylaxis and treatment of venous thrombosis and in the maintenance of anticoagulation in patients on warfarin who require surgery. For treatment and prophylaxis of thrombosis, the choice lies between unfractionated and low molecular weight (LMW) heparins e.g. Tinzaparin. In scenario 110, options B and D would provide comparable thromboprophylaxis but there is evidence that LMWH are associated with less bleeding in orthopaedic surgery and thus are preferable. LMWH also only require once daily injection and no routine monitoring of the coagulation screen is required.

Scenario 111 requires treatment of a confirmed venous thrombosis and either unfractionated on LMW heparins would be justified here. However the APTT ratio target range quoted in option C should be 1.5–2.5.

The patient in scenario 112 requires conversion to heparin to enable rapid changes to be made to his level of anti-coagulation peri-operatively. Although LMW heparins show more predictable bio-availability than unfractionated heparins, they have a longer half life and laboratory monitoring is less straightforward. Since the level of anti-coagulation is critical in this patient, most haematologists would advocate unfractionated heparin to maintain an APTT of 2.5–3.5.

Electrolyte disturbances

113. B   Fluid restriction
114. G   Haemofiltration
115. E   5% dextrose

The patient with the aortic aneurysm and chest infection is likely to have inappropriate ADH secretion. This can be confirmed by low plasma and urine osmolality. Chest infection is a known cause and the low serum sodium, relatively low urea and creatinine make this diagnosis likely. Excess ADH causes fluid retention and thus fluid restriction is appropriate.

The patient with sepsis has the classical electrolyte picture of acute renal failure. Hyponatraemia is commonly due to iatrogenic causes and poor excretion of the excess water. The renal failure here has not responded to volume loading or diuretics. Rising hyperkalaemia and anuria (particularly together) are indications for renal replacement therapy.

The child with the cerebral injury has neurogenic diabetes insipidus. Water is specifically lost and thus the serum sodium rises. The other minor abnormalities are due to haemoconcentration. Treatment involves fluid replacement with 5% dextrose i.e. 'dilution' is needed.

Respiratory physiology

116. A   Compliance
117. I   West's zones
118. B   Functional residual capacity
119. F FEV_1
120. H   Shunt
121. G   Dead space
122. J   Starling resistor
123. D   Vital capacity

The above definitions are self-explanatory. It is essential to have a thorough understanding of respiratory physiology and its terminology.

124.	Sum of CPP and ICP	C	Mean arterial blood pressure (MAP)
125.	Measures flow velocity in vessels	E	Transcranial Doppler sonography
126.	Global estimation of cerebral blood volume and oxygenation	F	Near-infrared spectroscopy
127.	Calculated from MAP and ICP	B	Cerebral perfusion pressure (CAP)

Secondary brain damage (after trauma, tumour or post-operatively, for instance) may be more destructive than the initial insult. It can be caused by hypoxia, or by cerebral ischaemia due to raised intracranial pressure, systemic hypotension, vasospasm, or other impairment of local perfusion. Information about cerebral haemodynamics at the cellular level is impossible to achieve and, in any case, is likely to vary considerably between different brain areas. The monitoring modalities listed above, allow only indirect assessment of the haemodynamic status of cerebral tissue, from which clinical judgements must be made.

60.   Spinal trauma   Answers:

128.	Flaccid areflexia, no anal tone, diaphragmatic breathing and priapism	H	Cervical cord injury
129.	Loss of position and vibration sensation	E	Left posterior column

The findings in the young man suggest a cervical cord injury as there is flaccid areflexia, flaccid anal sphincter and priapism.
The posterior columns carry proprioceptive impulses (two point discrimination and vibration nerve) from the same side of the body.

END OF CORE PAPER 2

CORE PAPER 3
SECTION 1 – MCQS

1. Metabolic response to injury   Answers: A C D E
The catabolic phase of the metabolic response to injury is accompanied by increased energy expenditure and a negative nitrogen balance. The size and duration of the response are directly related to the severity of the trauma or surgical insult.

2. Major burns   Answers: A B C D
Cardiovascular consequences of major burns may lead to excessive fluid loss causing haemodynamic compromise. Myocardial suppression from an associated myocardial depressant factor is also seen. Reduced RBC survival from increased capillary permeability and bone marrow depression occur. An initial thrombocytopenia followed by a later thrombocytosis is seen together with disseminated intravascular coagulation.

3. Blood volume   Answers: A B C
In response to hypovolaemia, baroreceptors in the carotid artery and aortic arch are stimulated. In addition, stretch receptors in the left atrium and pulmonary veins and juxta-glomerular apparatus are also stimulated. The resultant effect is a reduction in the flow of neural impulses from the baroreceptors to the brainstem so causing increased secretion of ADH. ADH release is stimulated by a decrease of 5–10% of the total circulating blood volume. In response to stress (i.e. hypovolaemia), there is increased release of adrenaline, cortisol and growth hormone, all of which increase blood glucose. Due to the action of corticosteroids and mineralocorticoids on the distal renal tubule, hypokalaemia may occur.

4. Renal blood flow   Answers: A B
At moderate systemic blood pressure (mean 80–160 mmHg) the renal vascular resistance adjusts blood pressure in the renal arterioles so that renal blood flow remains fairly constant (autoregulation). Hypertensive patients shift the range of autoregulation, thus they have a slightly reduced renal blood flow for a given blood pressure. Blood flow in the cortex is much higher than in the medulla. Autoregulation is impaired in shock, sepsis and low cardiac output states.

ANSWERS – Core Paper 3

151

5.   **Tracheostomy**   Answers: **B C D**

A tracheostomy is performed to relieve upper airway obstruction, to decrease dead space (achieves between 30 and 50% reduction), to assist ventilation and to facilitate bronchial toilet. Functional Residual Capacity (FRC) is the combination of the expiratory reserve volume and residual volume, of which the former is reduced following a tracheostomy.

6.   **Drugs and renal failure**   Answers: **A B D E**

Nephrotoxicity arises through several mechanisms: general and local vascular effects (diuretics, β-blockers, ACE inhibitors) or by direct tubular effects (proximal: aminoglycosides, radio-contrast, mannitol; distal: NSAIDs, ACE inhibitors, cyclosporin), tubular obstruction (sulphonamides, acyclovir), acute interstitial nephritis (β-lactams, vancomycin, ciprofloxacin, frusemide, thiazides) and acute glomerulonephritis (penicillamine). Frusemide is itself a nephrotoxic drug, but it may also be beneficial in renal failure. It reduces oxygen consumption and requirement in the medullary tubules of the kidney by inhibiting solute reabsorption and clearing tubular debris.

NSAIDs cause nephrotoxicity through several mechanisms: vasoconstriction within the renal circulation, reduction of medullary blood flow and oxygen delivery, alteration of potassium balance, inhibition of compensatory mechanisms protecting renal tubular blood flow in the volume depleted kidney. In addition, NSAIDs may cause an interstitial nephritis.

7.   **Regional blood flow**   Answers: **B D**

Cardiac output (heart rate x stroke volume) is the sum of the blood flow to all body regions and is dependent on body surface area. A Swan-Ganz catheter measures cardiac output by a thermodilution method (Fick principle) and it may be used to sample mixed venous blood, the oxygen saturation of which is also an indicator of cardiac output. If the cardiac output contains insufficient oxygen then anaerobic metabolism occurs with the formation of lactic acid. Neither cardiac output, blood lactate nor mixed venous oxygen saturation measure oxygen supply to a particular body region. Jugular bulb oxygen saturation is an indirect measurement of cerebral (i.e. regional) blood flow. Gastric tonometry measures anaerobic metabolism in the gastric mucosa and is an indirect measure of splanchnic (regional) blood flow.

8. Wound infection   Answers: A E

Local host factors predisposing to wound infection include prior irradiation in the field of the wound, the size of the bacterial inoculum, the presence of foreign bodies, tissue ischaemia, haematoma and seroma formation, tissue necrosis, the type and virulence of local organisms, and the pattern of resistance to antibiotics.

9. Suture materials   Answers: A B E

Non-absorbable sutures such as prolene may act as a nidus for concretion formation or sepsis if used in the renal tract. They are thus best avoided. Chromic catgut has an intracorporeal half-life of 10–14 days and should be avoided in the biliary tree as it may predispose to infection. No suture material has been shown to produce superior results for either small or large bowel anastomoses. Using the smallest calibre material strong enough to hold the tissues in question, minimising the amount of retained intracorporeal foreign body are sound surgical principles. The most commonly used suture material for bowel anastomoses include Vicryl, PDS and Maxon.

10. Skin grafts   Answers: C D E

Split skin grafts contain epidermis and varying amounts of dermis, and rely totally on the vascularity of the recipient site for survival. Thinner split grafts are more likely to 'take' than thicker ones because there is less tissue to be supported by imbibition. Lesser degrees of recipient site bacterial contamination, such as tissues containing $< 10^5$ organisms/mm^3, will usually allow a graft to 'take'.

11. Full thickness burns   Answers: A D E

Full thickness burns are pale, white or leathery, dry, and often have broken skin and exposed fat. They are painless and insensate due to thermal destruction of nerve endings.

12. ARDS   Answer: B

ARDS is initially due to pulmonary oedema of non-cardiac origin. Complement activation is the final common pathway independent of the causal factors. Aggregated neutrophils release superoxide radicals as a by-product of phagocytosis which may promote protein destruction (e.g. of collagen and elastin). There is increased shunting and associated pulmonary ventilation/perfusion mismatch. It is associated with diffuse pulmonary infiltrates on X-ray.

13.   Chest injuries   Answers: B C D

Although less than 10% of trauma admissions sustain cardiac or major vascular injury, thoracic trauma is responsible for 25% of trauma deaths. Most injuries (85%) can be managed without surgery. Tracheal rupture is an immediate threat to the airway and most people die before reaching hospital. A small number will reach hospital in a stable condition and undergo successful surgical repair.

14.   Lower chest wounds   Answers: A C

The diaphragm rises to the fourth intercostal space during full expiration, thus intra-abdominal viscera are at risk from penetrating lower chest wounds. 20% of lower chest stab wounds and 60% of lower chest gunshot wounds are associated with a significant intra-abdominal organ injury. Penetrating chest trauma requires chest drainage to deal with the associated pneumothorax and haemothorax.

15.   Critically injured patient   Answers: C D

A tension pneumothorax compromises ventilation and threatens life. It should be decompressed immediately using a needle or venflon inserted into the 2nd intercostal space in the mid-clavicular line. This must be followed by insertion of a chest drain.

Adequate ventilation requires adequate air exchange in addition to airway patency. If cardiovascular, respiratory, or neurological instability exists, ventilation should be accomplished with a bag-valve device to a mask or an endotracheal tube. Flail chest, tension pneumothorax, pulmonary contusion, open pneumothorax and haemothorax are frequently missed diagnoses that compromise ventilation. Endotracheal intubation, to secure a definitive safe airway, is indicated for unconscious patients and those with airway compromise due to mechanical factors. Cardiac tamponade may not give rise to distended neck veins if the patient is hypovolaemic. A narrow pulse pressure may be the only reliable sign.

16.   Neck trauma   Answers: A B D E

Signs of significant injury in penetrating neck trauma include an expanding haematoma, dysphonia, dysphagia and haemoptysis. Others include shock, external haemorrhage, reduced carotid pulsation, odynophagia, stridor, hoarseness, subcutaneous emphysema, lateralised neurological deficit, and a brachial plexus injury.

17.   Peritoneal lavage   Answers: A C E
Catheter aspiration of the normal uninjured peritoneal cavity may yield up to 5 ml of clear fluid. Lavage fluid exiting via a chest drain is an indicator of diaphragmatic injury and requires laparotomy. Accepted criteria for laparotomy on laboratory analysis of peritoneal lavage fluid (unspun) are > 100,000 RBCs/mm^3 or > 500 WBCs /mm^3.

18.   Traction injury   Answers: B C D
In Erb's palsy (traction injury of the upper roots and trunk – C5/6), there is paralysis of the abductors and lateral rotators of the shoulder, the elbow flexors and the supinator muscles. The arm hangs by the side medially rotated, extended at the elbow, and pronated. There is also loss of cutaneous sensation over the lateral aspect of the arm and forearm.

19.   Peroneal nerve   Answers: A C D E
The common peroneal nerve supplies the lateral and anterior muscular compartments of the calf and the skin over the anterior aspects of the calf and foot. With foot drop, the patient trips on walking as the toes catch the ground. Cutaneous innervation of the sole of the foot is through the medial and lateral plantar branches of the tibial nerve. Inversion is weakened because of paralysis of the tibialis anterior muscle. Muscle wasting is a sign of lower motor neurone damage. The peroneus longus tendon is one of the supports of the lateral arch; when paralysed the arch is compromised.

20.   Subdural haematoma   Answers: C E
Chronic subdural haematoma (CSH) is produced by rupture of veins passing from the cerebral hemispheres to the venous sinuses as a result of displacement of the brain inside the skull. It is bilateral in 50% cases. CSH may occur after only slight force and there may be no preceding loss of consciousness. Symptoms may not be apparent for weeks or months and can be undramatic (deteriorating mental capacity and mental slowness). Papilloedema is exceptional.

21.   Faecal occult blood test   Answers: C D
Faecal occult blood test screening with Haemoccult is a guaiac based test relying on a peroxidase-like reaction. Animal haemoglobin and certain vegetables containing peroxidase may give rise to false positives. FOBT has been shown to give a 15–30% reduction in incidence of colorectal cancer specific mortality in three different studies: Minnesota 33%; Nottingham 15%; and Funen (Denmark) 18% reduction in mortality. Approximately 10% of patients with a positive test will on investigation be shown to have a colorectal carcinoma.

22.   Breast cancer   Answers: C D E

Radical mastectomy and modified radical mastectomy have been shown to give the same results in terms of survival. Post-operative radiotherapy following either radical or modified radical mastectomy has not been shown to prolong the disease-free interval or survival, it only reduces the local recurrence rate. Conservative breast surgical management produces equivalent survival rates compared with more radical surgery.

23.   Oesophageal carcinoma   Answers: A C D

Pre-malignant lesions of the oesophagus include the Plummer-Vinson syndrome, corrosive oesophagitis, achalasia, Barrett's oesophagus, and scleroderma involvement of the oesophagus. There is a 25-fold increased risk of developing oesophageal cancer in Barrett's.

24.   Gastric cancer   Answers: A B E

A Krukenberg's tumour is a malignant deposit on the ovary associated with trans-coelomic tumour spread. It is common with gastric cancers. A Bloomer's shelf refers to a palpable pelvic tumour shelf on rectal examination resulting from intraperitoneal tumour spread. A Curling's ulcer is a acute stress gastroduodenal ulcer usually seen in burns patients. Courvoisier's sign refers to the axiom that a palpable gall bladder in the presence of jaundice is unlikely to be secondary to stones. A Virchow's node is an enlarged left supraclavicular lymph node resulting from tumour spread, and is common in gastric cancer. It may also be found in lung, breast, colon and pancreatic cancers.

25.   Carcinoid tumours   Answers: A B E

Carcinoid tumours of the colon and small bowel often behave in a malignant fashion, and often present with massive regional lymph node and hepatic metastases. The size of the primary tumour is a major prognostic factor. The carcinoid syndrome is due to the release of 5-HT and other hormonal peptides such as kallikrein into the systemic circulation. Therefore, malignant carcinoids of the gastrointestinal tract only produce carcinoid syndrome when metastases are present within the liver. 5-HIAA is the metabolite of 5HT and is excreted in increased amounts in the urine.

26.   Breast cancer   Answers: A B C D

Risk factors for the development of breast cancer include age > 45 years, nulliparity, contralateral breast cancer, family history of breast cancer, first full term pregnancy after 30 years of age, benign breast disease, early menarche and late natural menopause, and early artificial menopause.

27.   Blunt head trauma   Answers: A E

Duration of post traumatic amnesia (not retrograde amnesia) correlates well with primary brain injury. Blood alcohol levels correlate very poorly with degree of depression of conscious level in a patient with a head injury. The depression of conscious level must be assumed to be due to the head injury.

Adequate analgesia improves the cerebral perfusion pressure. Codeine phosphate does not interfere with pupillary reflexes. Haemodynamic stabilisation takes priority over evacuation of intracranial haematomas.

28.   Compartment syndrome   Answers: All false

Compartment syndrome may occur in the absence of a fracture. The diagnosis is clinical, although compartment pressure manometry may be useful in doubtful cases or unconscious patients. If pressures are being measured, fasciotomy should be performed when compartment pressure exceeds 40 mmHg. All compartments should be opened and the wounds should never be closed primarily. Delayed primary closure or split skin grafting may be performed once the swelling has settled.

29.   The oesophagus   Answer: A

The oesophagus is formed at the lower border of the cricoid cartilage. It is crossed anteriorly by the left main bronchus, lies behind the left atrium and passes through the muscular part of the diaphragm to the left of the central tendon through the muscular sling of the left crus. It is innervated in part by the recurrent laryngeal nerve, not the phrenic nerve.

30.   Left phrenic nerve   Answers: A B C D

The autonomic fibres in the phrenic nerve are sympathetic and pass from the superior (C1–4) and middle (C5/6) sympathetic cervical ganglia as grey rami into the C3–5 roots of the phrenic nerve, and innervate blood vessels in the diaphragm. The nerve lies on the fibrous pericardium and is sensory to the mediastinal and diaphragmatic pleura, and also to the diaphragmatic peritoneum. The phrenic nerve enters the chest by descending from the medial lower border of the scalenus anterior muscle between the subclavian vein anteriorly and artery posteriorly.

31.   Right lung   Answers: A C

Impressions on the mediastinal surface of the right lung include the trachea, vagus, superior vena cava, right atrium and subclavian artery. The oesophagus grooves the left lung above the arch of the aorta and below the hilum.

32.   **Clavipectoral fascia**   **Answers: D E**

The clavipectoral fascia is pierced by the cephalic vein and lateral pectoral nerve, overlain by the C4 dermatome (acromial branches of the supraclavicular nerves), and the infraclavicular lymph nodes. The fascia splits to enclose the pectoralis minor muscle, and continues beyond as the suspensory ligament of the axilla.

33.   **S1 nerve root compression**   **Answer: C**

Signs of S1 nerve root compression include reduced sensation in the S1 dermatome (sole of foot), weakness of plantar flexion of the ankle, and absent or reduced ankle jerk.

34.   **Asplenic patients**   **Answers: B C D**

Asplenic patients are at an increased risk of overwhelming sepsis caused by capsulated organisms such as *Streptococcus pneumoniae, Neisseria meningitidis,* and *Haemophilus influenza.* At present in the UK vaccination is recommended against Haemophilus and pneumococcus. It reduces the risk of infection and ideally should be given two weeks before surgery. Prophylactic oral antibiotics are effective at preventing post-splenectomy sepsis, which carries a 50% mortality. The antibiotic of choice is penicillin but erythromycin is indicated in cases of allergy.

35.   **Bacterial flora**   **Answers: C D E**

The predominant commensal bacteria of the skin is *Staphylococcus epidermidis.* Others include *Staphylococcus aureus,* micrococci, coryneforms and anaerobic cocci. The lower respiratory tract is usually sterile. The predominant bacterial flora of the oropharynx are *Streptococcus viridans,* coryneforms, and Neisseria. Many anaerobic bacteria colonise the colon, especially *Bacteroides fragilis.* The other main groups include clostridia. Aerobic bacteria such as *E. coli* and enterococcus are also present in large numbers. Lactobacilli are the predominant species in the vagina. Others include *Gardnerella vaginalis* and anaerobes.

36.   HIV infection   Answers: A B C

HIV is a retrovirus, and definitive diagnosis is made by Western blotting. More recently polymerase chain reaction techniques have been used. HIV is present in high titre in the blood of asymptomatic carriers, and in many asymptomatic HIV positive patients. The risk of seroconversion following a needlestick injury from an HIV positive patient is about 0.03%, and in a hepatitis B positive patient is about 30%. Hence, hepatitis B is potentially more infectious following a needlestick injury than HIV.

37.   Elective laparoscopic cholecystectomy   Answer: All false

Aspirin and warfarin reduce the risk of arterial emboli in atrial fibrillation. The International Normalised Ratio (INR) is a measure of Prothrombin Time (PT) and warfarin dosage should be adjusted to maintain the INR 1.5–2.5. Warfarin should be stopped before surgery as it predisposes to major haemorrhage, outweighing the risk of emboli. The risk of bleeding is small once the INR is less than 1.5. To prepare this patient for surgery, the warfarin should be stopped three days before scheduled surgery to allow the INR to fall to < 1.5. Generally aspirin does not need to be stopped before surgery. Warfarin could be recommenced after the operation once bleeding has stopped. For an elective operation as this, stopping the warfarin several days before the surgery and administering heparin or a low molecular weight heparin is the accepted course of management. The use of Vitamin K and FFP in this instance is wasteful of limited expensive resources.

38.   Raised mean cell volume   Answers: B C D E

A raised mean cell volume occurs with the macrocytosis associated with dietary deficiency or malabsorption of vitamins B_{12} and folate, liver disease, especially associated with alcohol abuse, hypothyroidism, myelodysplasia and after exposure to some drugs (cytotoxic, anti-HIV). Vitamin B_{12} is found exclusively in animal products and deficiency is a hazard of veganism. Conditions such as haemolytic anaemia or recovery from acute haemorrhage lead to an increased erythropoietic drive and hence the appearance of reticulocytes in the circulation. This may manifest as a raised mean cell volume because reticulocytes have a higher cell volume than mature red cells. Iron deficiency is associated with microcytosis.

39.   AB negative patient   Answers: A C D
The blood cells of an AB negative patient possess Landsteiner antigens A and B and the serum contains antibodies to the rhesus D antigen but not the A or B antigens. The patient may therefore receive any group of rhesus negative packed cells but can donate blood only to a rhesus positive or negative AB patient. Plasma products do not require cross-matching regardless of blood group.

40.   Sickle cell disease   Answers: B C E
Sickle cell disease results from a homozygous point mutation in the haemoglobin β-chain gene and may occur in patients of Afro-Caribbean, Arabic or Indian ethnic groups. Clinically, the disorder is characterised by chronic haemolysis. This may lead to production of pigment gallstones and also cause intermittent vaso-occlusive crises, severe musculo-skeletal pain, stroke, acute chest syndromes, mesenteric ischaemia, avascular necrosis of the femoral head and priapism. Splenic infarction is common, leading to splenic atrophy and functional hyposplenism. Increased peri-operative mortality arises from acute chest syndromes and stroke is precipitated by dehydration and inadequate oxygenation. Laboratory diagnosis is achieved by examination of the blood film and is confirmed by haemoglobin electrophoresis.

41.   Low molecular weight heparins   Answers: B C E
Low molecular weight heparins (LMWH) are prepared by enzymatic degradation of unfractionated heparin so reducing the mean molecular weight from 15 to 4–7 kD. LMWH therefore have a longer half-life than unfractionated heparin and better bioavailability after subcutaneous injection. Only once-daily administration is required. LMWH act predominantly by inhibiting Factor Xa and unlike unfractionated heparin, have low anti-thrombin activity. Consequently, a patient may be adequately anticoagulated with LMWH without prolongation of the APTT. Excretion is almost exclusively renal and so dose reduction is required in patients with renal failure.

42.   Warfarin   Answer: A
Warfarin is an orally active anticoagulant which rapidly depletes hepatic vitamin K by impairing its recycling. It acts by preventing the synthesis of the vitamin K dependent factors II, VII, IX and X, therefore it requires at least 48 hours to become effective. Although warfarin treatment will prolong both the APTT and the PT, the PT is a more reliable index of anticoagulant activity. It is usual practice to express the PT as an international normalised ratio (INR) when measuring anticoagulation. Complications of treatment include bleeding and rarely, skin necrosis. Warfarin has numerous interactions with other drugs, commonly antibiotics (either reducing or enhancing its bioavailability).

43.   Venous thrombosis   Answers: All true

Inherited deficiencies or defects in components of the coagulation cascade with anti-coagulant activity predispose to spontaneous and peri-operative venous thrombosis. These include antithrombin III, protein S and protein C deficiencies and the factor V Leiden mutation. Acquired risk rises with increasing age, malignancy, a previous history of thrombosis, immobilisation, obesity, the combined oral contraceptive pill, hormone replacement therapy and pregnancy. Thrombosis also occurs more frequently in patients with sickle cell disease, inflammatory bowel disease and myeloproliferative disorders.

44.   Red cell donations   Answers: A C E

All red cell donations in the United Kingdom are now screened for hepatitis B, hepatitis C, HIV-1, HIV-2 and *Treponema pallidum*. After screening, blood is not routinely subject to further manufacturing procedures to reduce the risk of infection transmission. Despite screening it is not possible to absolutely eliminate virally contaminated donor units because of the small proportion of false negative screening results and 'window periods' when donors may be viraemic yet have no serological response to infection. Organisms that may be transmitted by transfusion include: hepatitis A, human T-cell leukaemia viruses 1 and 2, cytomegalovirus, human parvovirus B19, *Treponema cruzii*, and malaria. Contamination of red cell donations by cold tolerant organisms such as Pseudomonas and *Yersinia enterocolitica* may lead to life-threatening sepsis in recipients.

45.   Transfusion reactions   Answers: B D E

Although acute haemolytic transfusions are almost exclusively due to ABO incompatibility, haemolysis may also occur due to anti-Rh D, Rh E, Rh C and anti-Kell antibodies. In these cases, haemolysis is within the liver and spleen. The usual presentation is fever, nausea and shivering usually about an hour after transfusion. Alternatively, in parous women or previous recipients of transfusions, there may be undetectable pre-transfusion antibodies which increase dramatically after re-exposure as a secondary antibody response. This may manifest as a delayed haemolytic transfusion reaction presenting 5–10 days after transfusion with fever, falling haemoglobin, jaundice and haemoglobinuria. Fever and rigors occur in about 1–2% of red cell and platelet transfusions and may indicate a non-haemolytic febrile transfusion reaction. This is most common in parous women and the previously transfused. It represents a recipient antibody response to donor white cell antigens. Allergic reactions ranging from mild urticaria to anaphylaxis are usually due to an antibody response to donor plasma proteins.

46.   Plasma substitutes   **Answers: B E**

Commonly used plasma substitutes include Dextran 40 and Dextran 70 (carbohydrates with average molecular weight 40,000 and 70,000 respectively) or alternatively partly degraded gelatin derivatives (Gelofusin® and Haemaccel®). The principal indication for these products is to expand and maintain plasma volume in conditions such as the acute phase of burns or septic shock. Shock due to sodium or water depletion is better treated with crystalloids. Acute volume expansion is hazardous in conditions such as congestive cardiac failure. Dextrans may interfere with crossmatching and some biochemical investigations.

47.   Statistical tests   **Answers: A B E**

t-tests and ANOVA (analysis of variance) are examples of parametric tests and can be used to assess Gaussian (normally) distributed data. The Wilcoxon and Mann-Whitney tests are non-parametric tests and are used for non-Gaussian data.

SECTION 2 – EMQs

Skin lesions

61. Malignant melanoma	D	S-100 positive on immunohisto-chemical staining
62. Basal cell carcinoma	E	Palisading basal cells at the periphery of tumour islands
63. Squamous cell carcinoma	B	Keratin pearl formation
64. Bowen's disease	C	Intra-epidermal (in situ) squamous carcinoma
65. Keratoacanthoma	A	Central keratin plug

Most cutaneous malignant melanomas stain S-100 positive using immunohistochemical techniques. Bowen's disease is an *in situ* SCC. Lesions occur as a reddened, scaly, slightly raised plaque. Invasion occurs only after many years, typically beyond 15–20 years. A keratoacanthoma is a self-limiting benign cutaneous tumour. A small red swelling grows quickly into a pale dome-shaped mass with a central keratin plug. These lesions regress spontaneously.

Histological tumour types

66. Villous adenoma	C	Neoplastic polyp
67. Peutz-Jeghers polyp	A	Hamartoma
68. Juvenile polyp	A	Hamartoma
69. Carcinoid tumour	B	Neuroendocrine tumour
70. Insulinoma	B	Neuroendocrine tumour
71. Leiomyosarcoma	D	Stromal tumour
72. Glucagonoma	B	Neuroendocrine tumour

Hamartomas resemble tumours but they are not neoplastic. They result from a localised disorder of the relationships of normal tissues, leading to over-production of one or more elements without the growth characteristics of tumours. Stromal cell tumours arise from smooth muscle or Schwann cells. They have different grades of malignancy and spectrum of aggressiveness. They are relatively radio-resistant and chemo-resistant.

Tumour markers

73.	Choriocarcinoma	B	β-hCG
74.	Hepatoma	A	α-fetoprotein
75.	Prostatic carcinoma	E	Acid phosphatase
76.	Colorectal cancer	C	Carcinoembryonic antigen
77.	Multiple myeloma	D	Paraproteins

Multiple myeloma is associated with the secretion of paraproteins which may be seen on an electrophoretic strip. Light chain protein (Bence-Jones) is secreted into the urine in myeloma. A proportion of colorectal carcinomas secrete carcinoembryonic antigen (CEA). CEA has a limited role in the follow-up of patients with colorectal cancer. Interpretation and intervention of late CEA rises remains controversial. Hepatomas may secrete α-fetoprotein, and teratomas β-hCG. Though not diagnostic, they have some role in screening investigation of tumours. They are useful for follow-up of recurrence. Acid phosphatase is now an uncommonly used marker of prostatic cancer, as it has a low specificity. Prostatic specific antigen is a much better tumour marker in terms of sensitivity and specificity.

Pathological chest conditions

78.	Mycelial mass with cellular debris	C	Aspergilloma
79.	Affects both visceral and parietal pleura	D	Malignant mesothelioma
80.	Connected to the airways and therefore contain air	A	Pulmonary cysts
81.	Is thought to have an autoimmune aetiology	E	Idiopathic mediastinal fibrosis
82.	Usually closely related to the trachea, hilum or oesophagus	B	Bronchogenic cysts

Bronchogenic cysts are congenital cysts of bronchial origin. They are usually closely related to the trachea, hilum of the lung or oesophagus. They usually present as an asymptomatic mass on CXR. Pulmonary cysts differ from bronchogenic cysts in that they are embedded in the pulmonary parenchyma. They are connected to the airways, and their walls do not contain cartilage.

An aspergilloma is the result of *aspergillus fumigatus* infection, which can cause an asthma-like condition or invasive lung infections. Malignant mesothelioma is asbestos-related and has a poor prognosis. It affects both parietal and visceral pleura. Idiopathic mediastinal fibrosis is due to diffuse collagenous fibrous replacement of the normal mediastinal connective tissue. It is thought to have an autoimmune aetiology.

Five year survival rates

83.	Carcinoid of the vermiform appendix	F	> 95%
84	Duke's A rectal cancer	E	80–90%
85.	Oesophageal cancer	B	5–10%
86.	Pancreatic carcinoma	A	< 5%
87.	Metastatic prostatic cancer	C	25%
88.	Duke's B rectal cancer	D	50–60%
89.	Carcinoid of the small bowel	D	50–60%

The overall 5-year survival rates of carcinoid tumours depend on the site of the primary. Those of the vermiform appendix have an approximate 98% 5-year survival, those of the small bowel and colon have an approximate 55% survival, and those of the rectum an 85% survival. The 5-year survival rates of Duke's A, B, and C rectal cancers are approximately 90%, 60%, and 30% respectively. Oesophageal and pancreatic cancer have a grave prognosis, and surgical cure is uncommon. Metastatic prostatic cancer can frequently be temporarily controlled by hormonal manipulation.

Cross matching of blood

90. C Crossmatched A rhesus D positive blood
91. D Uncrossmatched AB rhesus D positive blood
92. E Crossmatched AB rhesus D negative blood
93. A Uncrossmatched O rhesus D negative blood

This question relies on an understanding of two important principles:
(i) Antibodies against the A and B antigens are clinically significant and develop in everybody early in life according to their ABO blood group. Group A patients have anti-B antibodies and therefore cannot receive either B or AB blood. Similarly group B patients have anti-A antibodies and cannot receive A or AB blood. Group O patients have both anti-A and anti-B and can only receive group O blood and group AB patients have no anti-A or anti-B and can receive any blood.
(ii) Antibodies against rhesus D only develop in rhesus D negative patients after previous exposure to rhesus D positive red cells either during pregnancy or after a previous transfusion. Anti-rhesus D antibodies are usually clinically insignificant unless in pregnancy when they may lead to rhesus haemolytic disease of the newborn in rhesus D positive infants.

In scenarios 90 and 92 both patients have the same ABO and rhesus D type. In scenario 92 however, the rhesus D negative female patient is of childbearing age and so it is essential that she receives rhesus D negative blood and should if possible receive ABO compatible blood. The patient in scenario 90 is unlikely to encounter any ill effects from receiving rhesus D positive blood and since AB rhesus D negative blood is extremely uncommon it is quite reasonable to administer group A blood which is ABO compatible. Both patients require elective transfusion so should receive fully crossmatched blood.

The patients in scenarios 91 and 93 both require an emergency transfusion which justifies the use of uncrossmatched blood. However, since the patient in scenario 91 has been recently 'group and saved' it is possible to administer ABO rhesus D identical blood. If the ABO and rhesus D groups are unknown, it is justifiable to administer O rhesus D negative blood which is unlikely to provoke a severe transfusion reaction whatever the group of the recipient.

Blood gas data interpretation

94. F   Acetylsalicylic acid overdose
95. D   Cardiorespiratory arrest, during resuscitation
96. B   Vomiting and fluid loss from biliary fistula
97. A   Tachypnoea, accessory muscles of respiration, intercostal recession
98. C   IDDM with pneumonia
99. G   24 hours after major crush injury

In the early stages, aspirin overdose classically produces a respiratory alkalosis due to hyperventilation. Vomiting and bile loss produces a hypochloraemic metabolic alkalosis. A diabetic may become acidotic when ill, and pneumonia produces hypoxia. A cardiac arrest produces a mixed respiratory and metabolic acidosis The high pO_2 is probably because the patient is being ventilated with 100% oxygen during resuscitation. The hyperkalaemia seen after crush injuries is due to the massive release of intracellular potassium following tissue destruction.

Renal failure

100. D   Intravenous or nebulised salbutamol
101. A   0.9% saline
102. C   Dopamine

A potassium of 7.4 mmol/l is potentially life threatening. The best option here is to administer salbutamol, which acts like insulin (usually given with dextrose in this situation), by increasing potassium uptake into cells. However, salbutamol is much safer (no hypoglycaemia) and is quicker to prepare. Definitive treatment will subsequently be required.
CSF contains large amounts of sodium and unless replaced with fluid of adequate sodium concentration (0.9% saline) total body sodium may be depleted.
The final case demonstrates inadequate perfusion. The CVP is markedly elevated and the patient has excess intravascular volume due to poor cardiac function. Thus, an inotrope will be required to improve cardiac (pump) function.

Bleeding in an anti-coagulated patient

103. D Intravenous phytomenadione and fresh frozen plasma 30 ml/kg
104. F Intravenous protamine sulphate

Scenario 103. is a common clinical problem in which a patient who has been stable on warfarin for some time becomes over-anticoagulated because the co-prescription of antibiotics has impaired hepatic metabolism of warfarin. Life-threatening bleeding is treated with a slow intravenous infusion of 5 mg phytomenadione (vitamin K) and fresh frozen plasma. Intramuscular phytomenadione should be avoided as it has poor bioavailability and is likely to cause a haematoma. Less severe haemorrhage may require 0.5–2 mg of phytomenadione intravenously and withdrawal of warfarin until the INR returns to the normal range. Elevation of the INR without bleeding may just require cessation of anticoagulation and observation.

Scenario 104 requires urgent heparin neutralisation with intravenous protamine sulphate (maximum 50 mg). 1 mg of protamine neutralises 100 units of heparin. Since the half-life of heparin is short, less severe bleeding may be safely treated by cessation of heparin and observation.

Trauma due to RTA

105.	Pelvic and acetabular fractures	B	Side impact RTA
106.	Myocardial contusion	A	Frontal impact RTA
107.	Lateral flail chest	B	Side impact RTA
108.	Aortic transection	A	Frontal impact RTA
109.	Lower limb fractures	D	Pedestrian in an RTA

Different mechanisms of injury give rise to different related injury patterns, though there is much overlap between each. Frontal impact is more likely to produce cervical spine fractures, anterior flail chest, myocardial contusion, pneumothorax, aortic transection, and liver/spleen rupture. Side impact is more likely to produce cervical spine fractures, lateral flail chest, pneumothorax, pelvic and acetabular fractures, and liver/spleen rupture. Rear impact is more likely to produce cervical spine injury. Pedestrians in RTAs are likely to suffer head injury, thoracic and abdominal injuries, and fractures of the lower limbs (e.g. tibial plateau fractures).

Intracranial haemorrhage/thrombosis

110.E Internal carotid artery
111.C Middle meningeal artery
112.F Cerebral vein
113.H Cerebral artery
114.A Cavernous venous sinus

- Expanding internal carotid artery aneurysms in the cavernous sinus can erode into the sphenoidal air sinus medially and also compress the lateral wall of the cavernous sinus damaging III, IV, Va, and Vb. VI is most commonly involved as it passes through the venous sinus in the adventitia of the artery. Rupture of the aneurysm into the cavernous sinus creates a carotid-cavernous sinus fistula; blood may dissect through the eroded passage medially into the sphenoid air sinus from whence it drains through the sphenoethmoidal recess into the nasal cavity, relieving the pressure in the sinus. In this case, only VI is affected giving diplopia and a medial strabismus. Diplopia is worse on looking to the left as abduction is paralysed in the affected eye.

- This is a typical history of a developing extradural haematoma from a middle meningeal artery bleed after skull fracture at the pterion. The lucid interval is extended because the bleed is contained between the meningeal and endosteal layers of the dura mater, which are dissected apart as the bleed progresses.

- This is a typical history of a subdural haematoma after tearing a cerebral vein as it lies in the subdural space above the arachnoid mater at the point of entry into the superior sagittal sinus. The tear occurs by shearing at the vein/sinus interface, when a forward accelerating movement of the head is suddenly arrested. Movement of the skull and associated dural sinuses are halted, but the forward movement of the brain and cerebral veins continues. The lucid interval is protracted because of the low and often negative pressures in the system.

- This is a typical history of a massive subarachnoid haemorrhage, in this case, from a ruptured large cerebral artery aneurysm. The lucid period is short and commonly absent altogether. Intracranial pressure quickly builds and, unless relieved, death rapidly ensues.

- Cavernous sinus thrombosis may result from the spread of infection from areas drained by the venous tributaries of the sinus, in this case, ophthalmic veins draining the chronically infected ethmoidal air sinuses. There is oedema of all drainage areas and resulting exophthalmos. Complete ophthalmoplegia may ensue as III, IV and VI become involved. Damage to Va (and Vb) causes severe pain over cutaneous distributions.

Anatomy of thorax

115. Inferior vena cava	G	Recurrent laryngeal nerve
116. Bifurcation of the brachio-cephalic artery	C	Right pulmonary artery
117. Oblique fissure of the right lung	E	4th rib
118. Left ventricle	A	5th intercostal space
119. Hilum of the lung	H	3rd intercostal space
120. Commencement of the superior vena cava	F	1st left costal cartilage
121. Lower border of the arch of the aorta	D	Manubriosternal joint
122. Termination of the thoracic duct	C	Right pulmonary artery

When reading X-rays and examining patients the following are some of the important landmarks:

1. The inferior vena cava passes through the diaphragm at the vertebral level of T8.

2. The brachiocephalic artery bifurcates behind the right sterno-clavicular joint behind the commencement of the right brachio-cephalic vein (confluence of the right subclavian and right internal jugular veins).

3. The oblique fissure of the right lung passes along the line of the right 4th rib from the right mid-clavicular line to the right sternal margin.

4. The left ventricle lies behind the left 5th intercostal space from the left sternal margin to the left mid-clavicular line.

5. The hilum of each lung lies behind the 3rd and 4th costal cartilages and intervening 3rd intercostal space, on each side.

6. The commencement of the superior vena cava (confluence of the left and right brachiocephalic veins) lies behind the lower border of the right costal cartilage.

7. The lower border of the arch of the aorta bisects the trans-thoracic plane, the surface marking of which is the sternal angle.

8. The thoracic duct drains into the left brachiocephalic vein at its commencement (confluence of the left subclavian and left internal jugular veins) – all these structures lie behind the left sterno-clavicular joint.

ANSWERS – Core Paper 3

Local anaesthetic agents

123. Commonly used for conjunctival anaesthesia	B	Amethocaine
124. Caused several deaths when used in Bier's blocks	A	Bupivacaine
125. Causes sympathetic stimulation	D	Cocaine
126. Is the best agent for Bier's blocks	C	Prilocaine
127. Is formulated with hyperbaric phenol	G	None of above

Amethocaine is an ester which rapidly diffuses into the conjunctiva. Cocaine is also an ester but causes sympathetic stimulation and so is reserved for situations where vasoconstriction is required (e.g. nasal procedures). All the other local anaesthetics are amides. Bupivacaine binds to the myocardium and has caused a number of deaths when used in Bier's blocks. Thus, it is now contraindicated for use in Bier's blocks. Prilocaine binds poorly to the myocardium and so is the best agent for intravenous regional anaesthesia. Hyperbaric solutions are produced by the inclusion of 8% dextrose. Phenol is very neurotoxic and is not routinely formulated with any of the local anaesthetic agents.

END OF CORE PAPER 3

1.   **Inotropes**   Answers: C E

α_1 receptor stimulation leads to vasoconstriction. β_1 receptors are located in the heart and stimulation leads to increased heart rate and contractility. β_2 receptor stimulation dilates peripheral and coronary arteries and arterioles.

Noradrenaline is a very potent α_1 agonist and has some β_1 agonist activity. It is more efficient than adrenaline for increasing blood pressure.

Adrenaline stimulates both α and β receptors. At higher doses, adrenaline causes vasoconstriction.

Dobutamine is a predominantly β_1 receptor agonist. It exerts a more prominent inotropic than chronotropic action.

Isoprenaline is a pure β_2 receptor agonist that has a more chronotropic action and is used to speed up the heart in patients where pacing is impractical. It is a temporising measure.

Dopexamine is a synthetic analogue of dopamine, with the theoretical advantage of having dopaminergic activity without α effects. It causes splanchnic and renal vasodilatation.

2.   **Shock**   Answers: A C E F

Changes in cellular metabolism associated with shock include accumulation of lactic acid and reduced ATP production due to anaerobic metabolism. Changes in membrane function result in passage of sodium into cells and passage of potassium out of cells. Lysosomal fragmentation occurs as a result of autodigestion. Fatty acid mobilisation results in increased ketone production.

3.   **Hyperbaric oxygen therapy**   Answers: A C D

Hyperbaric oxygen is an oxygen tension of significantly greater than 1 atmosphere. An anaesthetic breathing circuit can only achieve approximately 1 atmosphere, so a pressurised chamber is required. Typically treatment involves several sessions of an hour or more. Indications include treatment of gas gangrene, necrotising fasciitis and carbon monoxide poisoning. Exposure to more than 2 atmospheres tension of oxygen may cause acute oxygen toxicity which is manifested by convulsions.

4.   Squamous cell carcinoma   Answers: All true

Squamous cell carcinoma is the second most common cutaneous malignancy (the commonest is basal cell carcinoma). It may arise in an area of Bowen's disease and predisposing factors include exposure to sun, radiation, certain chemicals and albinism. Squamous cell carcinoma is locally invasive and treatment involves excision with block dissection of draining nodes, if they are involved. Squamous cell carcinomas also respond to radiotherapy and early lesions can be treated topically with 5 fluorouracil.

5.   Pancreatic biopsy   Answers: B C D

Kocherisation of the duodenum aids trucut biopsy of the pancreatic head but is not mandatory. Open wedge biopsy is suitable at laparotomy and is generally more accurate than other methods. FNA cytology can provide a definitive diagnosis of malignancy, but requires skilled cytologists. Pancreatic biopsy has an overall complication rate of <10%. Sepsis, bleeding, and fistula formation are common complications.

6.   Basal cell carcinomas   Answers: B C D F G H

Epidermoid carcinoma is an alternative name for a squamous cell carcinoma. BCC (rodent ulcer) is associated with sunlight exposure. Local invasion of bone/cartilage only occurs in neglected cases of BCC, and metastases are exceedingly rare. BCCs commonly recur locally because they are often multifocal, occurring in an area of field change.

7.   ARDS   Answer: C

The clinical diagnosis is usually provided by a history of a catastrophic pulmonary event (e.g. aspiration or pulmonary sepsis), respiratory failure, (exclusion of cardiogenic pulmonary oedema or chronic lung disease as the cause of respiratory failure), and diffuse pulmonary infiltrates on X-ray. Lung biopsy is not required. In ARDS, the lung is stiffer and therefore pulmonary compliance is reduced. The overall mortality is approximately 50%. Prognosis is dependent on the age of the patient, the presence of other organ complications, and the severity of the lung injury.

8.   Cardiac tamponade   Answers: A D

The classical triad of symptoms of cardiac tamponade (Beck's triad) includes muffled heart sounds, distended neck veins and pulsus paradoxus. Pulsus paradoxus is defined as a fall in systolic blood pressure by > 10 mmHg with inspiration. In cardiac tamponade, the cardiac outline is classically globular shaped on CXR. Charcot's triad refers to fever, jaundice and abdominal pain, and is suggestive of ascending cholangitis.

ANSWERS – Core Paper 4

9. Diaphragmatic rupture   **Answer: C**

Traumatic diaphragmatic rupture following blunt trauma occurs most commonly on the posterolateral aspect of the left hemi-diaphragm. The initial CXR changes are usually non-specific. DPL is insensitive for diaphragmatic injury.

10. Fibroadenomas   **Answers: A B D**

Fibroadenomas of the breast arise from breast lobules rather than ducts. They contain both epithelial and stromal elements. There is a very slight increased risk of cancer development in patients with fibroadenomas (cystosarcoma phylloides tumours may arise in pre-existing fibro-adenomas). Up to 40% of fibroadenomas spontaneously regress or resolve. They do not usually interfere with breast feeding.

11. Gastric cancer   **Answers: All true**

Approximately 95% of gastric cancers are adenocarcinomas, with about 4% being lymphomas and 1% leiomyosarcomas. Predisposing factors include previous partial gastrectomy (this probably relates to chronic achlorhydria) blood group A, chronic atrophic gastritis, gastric polyps and *Helicobacter pylori* infection. Anorexia and weight loss occur in > 95% of cases. Pyloric obstruction occurs mainly with distal lesions. Dysphagia occurs with proximal lesions. About half present with a palpable abdominal mass.

12. Faecal occult blood testing   **Answers: A C E**

Faecal occult blood testing with Haemoccult requires up to 20 ml of blood to be passed in the stool per day before being reliably positive. It has a sensitivity of 10% in detecting large adenomatous polyps, and 50–70% for colon cancer. These figures reflect the intermittent nature of bleeding in both scenarios. Upper GI bleeding is less likely to be detected than colonic bleeding because the peroxidase-like activity is reduced as haemoglobin travels through the gut.

13. Viral hepatitis   **Answers: B C D**

Hepatitis B can be vertically transmitted from mother to baby and is the most important means of transmission world-wide. The e antigen is produced in excess during viral replication and its detection indicates a high degree of infectivity. The surface antigen is found in acute hepatitis and persists in chronic carriers.

14.   Actinomycosis   Answers: D

Actinomycetes are Gram-positive microaerophilic bacteria, present as part of the normal flora of the mouth, lower gut, and female genital tract. It is therefore an endogenous infection. The commonest site of actinomycosis infection is cervicofacial, occurring in about 50% of cases. Other sites of infection include the abdomen, thorax, and female genital tract. The commonest organism producing infection is *Actinomyces israelii*, though *Actinomyces propionica* is occasionally responsible. Culture of the organism is slow, taking a week or more to produce positive cultures. The discharge contains characteristic sulphur granules.

15.   Pulmonary tuberculosis   Answers: C F G

Mycobacterium tuberculosis hominis is the commonest causal organism of pulmonary tuberculosis in humans, and is usually spread by air droplets. *Mycobacterium tuberculosis bovis* predominantly causes gastrointestinal tuberculosis, and is usually spread by ingestion of infected milk. The hypersensitivity reaction is mediated by T-lymphocytes, which liberate lymphokines. The Gohn focus refers to the initial site of infection in a non-immune individual. It is usually subpleural in location in the well aerated portions of the lung (the upper lobe and upper part of the lower lobe).

16.   Disseminated candidiasis   Answers: B D

Blood cultures are negative in up to 80% of cases of disseminated candidiasis. Ophthalmitis is one of the diagnostic criteria of disseminated candidiasis. Gastro-intestinal candidiasis may be treated with nystatin as it is not absorbed from the gut. However, the drug of choice in disseminated disease is amphotericin B. Predisposing factors include antibiotic therapy, steroids, leucopenia and immunosuppressed states. Death rates are higher in neutropenic patients.

17.   Severely injured patients   Answers: A B D

Blood loss is a leading cause of death in severely injured patients and hypotension must be assumed to be hypovolaemic in origin until proven otherwise. Loss of 50% or more of blood volume leads to a critical impairment in cerebral perfusion and results in loss of consciousness. Tourniquets produce anaerobic metabolism and increase blood loss if incorrectly applied. They may also result in limb ischaemia. A high-riding prostate may indicate significant urethral injury and is a contraindication to urethral catheterization. A urethrogram is used to assess urethral integrity. Neck wounds penetrating through the platysma require surgical evaluation, and may require pre-operative investigations such as arteriography, bronchoscopy, oesophagoscopy and Gastrografin swallow.

18.   Tension pneumothorax   Answers: B C D

Tension pneumothorax produces acute severe respiratory embarrassment in association with profound hypotension, absence of breath sounds on the affected side, hyper-resonance to percussion on the affected side, distended neck veins, and tracheal deviation to the opposite side.

19.   Hepatobiliary trauma   Answers: B D

Pringle's manoeuvre refers to occlusion of the hepatic artery and portal vein by compression of the free edge of the lesser omentum. It is used to control major haemorrhage from liver trauma. Penetrating hepatic trauma is usually associated with localised injury. Blunt trauma often causes severe disruption of intra-hepatic bile ducts and vessels, devitalisation of tissues, and carries a higher mortality than penetrating trauma. Devitalised hepatic tissue should be excised and drainage provided. There is no evidence that gallstone spillage is a major cause of late sepsis.

20.   Peritoneal lavage   Answers: B

The only absolute contraindication to DPL is any existing indication for laparotomy. DPL under these circumstances would not alter management decisions, and would only delay transfer to theatre and subsequent correction of potentially life-threatening injuries. Relative contraindications include advanced pregnancy, advanced cirrhosis, previous abdominal operations, morbid obesity, and established pre-existing coagulopathy.

21.   Thoracic and lumbar spine injuries   Answer: B

Thoracic spine fractures are commonly multiple, particularly in the lower thoracic spine. The thoracic paraspinal line should normally be about one-third of the width of the descending aorta. On plain X-rays it is often impossible to differentiate simple wedge fractures of the lumbar spine from burst fractures with fragments impinging on the cord. Oblique thoracic spine X-rays rarely add any information. A CT would be the best imaging modality. On the AP lumbar spine film, the interpedicular distance should gradually widen from L1 to L5.

22.   Spinal injuries   **Answer: B**

Intravenous methylprednisolone 30 mg/kg initially then 5.4 mg/kg/hour for 23 hours has been shown to improve neurological recovery. Other treatments such as naloxone and mannitol have not. Unstable thoracic spine fractures can safely be treated by maintaining the spine in the neutral position ('postural reduction'). Although many centres operate early to allow early mobilization, there is no evidence that this improves neurological recovery.

Fractures of the pedicles of C2 (the 'hangman's fracture') are unstable fractures in which the cord is put at risk by distraction. They should initially be treated by in line immobilization.

The initial neurological examination is a poor predictor of prognosis as spinal shock can mimic complete cord injury.

23.   Malignant breast tumours   **Answers: A D**

Mammographic features suggestive of a malignant tumour include localised spiculated microcalcification of variable density, a dense lesion of stellate appearance, and a poorly circumscribed lesion of increased density.

24.   Colorectal cancer   **Answers: B D**

Adjuvant chemotherapy has been shown to produce a modest survival advantage in Duke's C and some Duke's B colorectal cancers. The best results have been with 5-FU administered alone or in combination with folinic acid (leucovorin).

25.   Tamoxifen   **Answers: A D E**

Tamoxifen is a cytostatic and immunomodulatory drug that selectively binds to oestrogen receptors on breast cancer cells. It is very well tolerated, though 5–10% of women have side-effects that include flushes, nausea, weight gain, vaginal dryness and bleeding. A four fold increase in endometrial cancer has been described in patients taking a five year course of tamoxifen. The usual dose for first-line adjuvant treatment is 20 mg/day. In addition to its effects on an existing breast cancer, tamoxifen appears to reduce the incidence of contralateral breast cancers (13% at 1 year, 47% at 5 years), myocardial infarction and osteoporosis.

26.   Major burns   **Answers: B D**

Major burns are associated with splanchnic vasoconstriction on both the arteriolar and venular sides of the circulation. Curling's are stress ulcers related to major burns. They have a propensity to massive bleeding and have a poor prognosis.

27.   Soft tissue coverage   Answers: A C E

Composite grafts include skin, subcutaneous tissue, and other tissue elements such as cartilage. They are free grafts and rely on imbibition and diffusion. Therefore, they are size-limited. Human epithelial cells can be cultured to provide sheets for grafting. From a biopsy of 4 cm^2, up to 2 m^2 can be grown in three weeks. This is useful for large burns. Autografts last long-term. Free flaps generally rely on blood supply from an artery of least 1 mm in diameter, with microvascular anastomosis to restore blood supply. Advancement flaps depend on the laxity of their skin to provide excess tissue when separated from their underlying structures. They are useful when the skin is excessive and has a good blood supply, such as in the ageing face.

28.   Coronary artery bypass surgery   Answers: A D

The patency rate of internal mammary artery grafts is approximately 90% at 10 years. Vein grafts anastomosed at the same locations have a 10-year patency rate of only about 40%. A major factor predictive of outcome is left ventricular function, and this is thought to be more important than the age of the patient or the number of grafts performed. Predictive risk scores are used in cardiac surgery (e.g. Parsonnet) to give an estimated risk. The score is based on age, ejection fraction, previous CVA, number of diseased vessels, diabetes mellitus etc. Failure of internal mammary graft function is usually a technical problem and occurs early. Long-term failure of vein grafts is due to intimal proliferation and atheroma deposition.

29.   Laser surgery   Answers: B D

Laser surgery uses monochromatic light of intense energy, which liberates heat on contact with tissues. It can cut, coagulate or vaporise tissues. It poses potential danger to patients' and operators' eyes and requires the use of safety glasses and non-reflective instruments. The effects of laser depend on absorption and scatter, which are related to the tissue type, colour, and specific pigments present. High energy can be focused onto a small lesion, and allows precision causing little surrounding tissue damage.

30.   Lateral hemi-section of L5 cord   Answers: B E

L5 cord lesions cause ipsilateral loss of fine touch and contralateral loss of pain and temperature sensation below the lesion. There is an ipsilateral upper neurone lesion with brisk reflexes, a Babinski sign, but no muscle wasting.

31.   Brachiocephalic vein   Answers: A C D E
The left brachiocephalic vein drains blood from the cervical vertebrae via both vertebral veins, the thyroid gland by the inferior thyroid veins, the first left intercostal space via the left superior intercostal veins, and all anterior intercostal spaces by anterior intercostal veins draining into the internal thoracic veins. The thoracic duct enters the vein at its commencement behind the left sternoclavicular joint. The bronchial veins drain into the azygos/hemiazygos systems.

32.   Middle lobe of right lung   Answers: C D
The middle lobe of the right lung has two bronchopulmonary segments and is separated from the lower lobe by the oblique fissure. It is auscultated in the 5th intercostal space anteriorly (the lower lobe intervenes posteriorly). Both the right atrium and the dome of the diaphragm make large impressions on the lung surface.

33.   The diaphragm   Answers: B C D E
The left crus is attached to the L1/2 vertebrae, and both crura are pierced by the sympathetic splanchnic nerves. Inferior phrenic arteries (the first branches of abdominal aorta) supply the diaphragm and both suprarenal glands lie against the diaphragm retroperitoneally. Both kidneys lie on the lateral arcuate ligaments and thus a pneumothorax is a possible complication of nephrectomy.

34.   The breast   Answers: A B D
The blood supply to the breast is mainly derived from the lateral thoracic artery. The internal thoracic artery, perforating intercostal arteries and the pectoral branches of the thoracoabdominal artery also contribute to the arterial supply of the breast. Venous return simply follows the arteries mentioned above. 75% of the lymph drains through the axillary nodes, and the retro-mammary space overlies the pectoralis major muscle. The nipple is a reliable marker for the T4 dermatome.

35.   Foramen magnum   Answers: A B C E
The structures passing through the foramen magnum include: medulla oblongata and meninges, spinal parts of the accessory nerves, the meningeal branches of the upper cervical nerves, vertebral arteries, anterior and posterior spinal arteries.

36.   Haemolytic anaemia   Answers: B C

The laboratory findings in haemolytic anaemia include the biochemical markers of increased red cell breakdown: unconjugated hyperbilirubinaemia, increased excretion of urobilinogen in the urine and stercobilinogen in the faeces. Haptoglobins normally eliminate free haemoglobin in the plasma and in haemolysis they characteristically become saturated and are absorbed by reticuloendothelial cells. Hyperbilirubinaemia may lead to pigment gallstones. Increased red cell turnover leads to marrow hyperplasia and increased production of reticulocytes, hence leading to an increased mean cell volume.

37.   Sickle cell disease   Answer: D

The mainstay of the peri-operative management of patients with sickle cell disease is the prevention of vaso-occlusive crises with adequate hydration and oxygenation. Functional hyposplenism increases the risk of post-operative sepsis and appropriate broad spectrum antibiotic prophylaxis should accompany all procedures. Heparin anticoagulation is advisable because of the increased risk of thrombosis. Baseline haemoglobin concentrations in sickle cell disease may be 6–7 g/dl and 'over-transfusion' to 14 g/dl increases the risk of vaso-occlusive events. Pre-operative exchange transfusion aims to reduce the proportion of haemoglobin S to < 30% of total haemoglobin without an increase in the overall haemoglobin concentration. This is usual for most procedures except for those involving very brief periods of general anaesthesia when no intervention is required.

38.   Aspirin   Answer: A

Aspirin is an irreversible inhibitor of platelet cyclo-oxygenase and therefore reduces platelet thromboxane A2 (which usually promotes platelet aggregation and local vasoconstriction). Its main use is in the prevention of arterial thrombosis which is more critically dependent on platelet activation and aggregation than venous thrombosis. Patients who have received aspirin continue to show impaired platelet function until the platelet pool has been replaced from the marrow and therefore aspirin should be discontinued at least seven days before surgery for its full anti-thrombotic effects to be eliminated. Aspirin is orally active and carries with it the risk of upper gastrointestinal haemorrhage but very seldom bleeding at other sites.

39.   Coagulation factors   Answers: B C D E

Coagulation is initiated in vivo by the interaction between tissue factor (TF) in the tissues and factor VII in the plasma. Anatomical separation of TF from the plasma prevents activation of the pathway unless vascular integrity is breached. Alternatively, coagulation can be initiated if there is pathological expression of TF on vascular cells as in malignancy, disseminated intravascular coagulation and inflammation. If TF and Factor VII interact, the resultant complex activates factor X and so completes the extrinsic pathway. Factor X in turn activates small quantities of thrombin which back activates Factors V, VIII, IX and X (intrinsic and common pathways) in the presence of anionic phospholipids on the surface of activated platelets. This provides amplification of the pathway by generating larger quantities of thrombin. Eventually sufficient thrombin is formed to cleave fibrinogen to fibrin to form a thrombus. Coagulation is limited *in vivo* by the activation of the anticoagulants antithrombin III, protein S and protein C by thrombin.

40.   Disseminated intravascular coagulation   Answers: D E

Disseminated intravascular coagulation (DIC) is a multisystem disorder characterised by simultaneous activation of the coagulation and fibrinolytic pathways. Common causes include sepsis, malignancy (especially adenocarcinoma), trauma and obstetric emergencies (e.g. placenta abruption, amniotic fluid embolism). Although DIC usually manifests as bleeding, some patients display thrombosis. Progressive consumption of all the coagulation factors and platelets leads to a characteristic laboratory profile of prolongation of the PT, APTT and TT and falling fibrinogen and platelets. Increased fibrinolysis is indicated by rising concentrations of fibrinogen degradation products or D-dimers. Although similar findings may be a feature of hepatic insufficiency, DIC may be diagnosed by demonstrating deteriorating coagulation abnormalities in conjunction with a likely clinical cause. The mainstay of care is treatment of the underlying cause, replacement of the deficient factors with fresh frozen plasma, cryoprecipitate and platelets.

41. Platelet transfusion   Answers: All false

Most haematologists now recommend that pre-operative platelet transfusion should only be administered if the count is $< 100 \times 10^9/l$ for neurological and ophthalmic surgery, $< 80 \times 10^9/l$ for most other surgical procedures, lumbar puncture or liver biopsy, $< 50 \times 10^9/l$ for minor procedures such as central venous catheterization. These guidelines should be relaxed if there is an additional haemostatic defect or in the event of bleeding. Patients not requiring imminent surgery do not require platelet transfusion unless the count is $< 10 \times 10^9/l$ as spontaneous bleeding is unlikely. Transfused platelets have a short half-life *in vivo*. It should be given as close to surgery as practicable and given as often as indicated by the clinical state. Patients with immune thrombocytopenia will have a very poor response to transfused platelets and attempts to increase the platelet count before splenectomy should be performed with corticosteroids or intravenous immunoglobulin before resorting to platelet transfusion.

42. Peri-operative transfusion   Answer: D

Although it is popularly believed that all patients with a pre-operative haemoglobin of < 10 g/dl should be transfused, clinical studies show that cardiac output does not increase sharply until the haemoglobin falls well below 7 g/dl. Young patients tolerate haemodilution well, especially women. For acute peri-operative blood loss of less than 20% of total blood volume, resuscitation with a suitable crystalloid is usually sufficient unless there is a contraindication. In the elderly, pre-existing cardio-respiratory disease is much more likely and more aggressive transfusion is usually required, although rapid transfusion is unwise because of the risk of volume overload. Total blood volume is approximately 70 ml/kg in adults and 80 ml/kg in children.

43. Massive blood transfusion   Answers: B C D

Complications associated with massive blood transfusion include hyperkalaemia, hypothermia (blood is stored at 4°C, fast flow blood warmers may reduce the hypothermia and should be used routinely), disseminated intravascular coagulation, thrombocytopenia (dilutional – stored blood is low in functional platelets), and hypocalcaemia (due to citrate in stored blood).

44.   Digoxin   Answer: D
Digoxin suppresses conduction through the atrio-ventricular node reducing the rate of ventricular contraction in atrial fibrillation and flutter, but does not convert atrial fibrillation or flutter to sinus rhythm. Digoxin has no place in the treatment of ventricular fibrillation, which requires electrical defibrillation. Digoxin has a therapeutic index of 2 (i.e. low) and the toxicity is exacerbated by hypokalaemia. It is not known to alter the effects of warfarin.

45.   Statistical analysis   Answer: D
The p-value is a probability with a value ranging from zero to one. The threshold p-value for significance is traditionally set at 0.05. If one compares two means, the null hypothesis is that the two populations have the same means. A p-value of 0.001 is more significant than a p-value of 0.01. The smaller the p-value, the more significant the result.

46.   Acute haemolytic transfusion reaction   Answers: A B D E
The other features of acute haemolytic transfusion reaction include pyrexia, flushing, lumbar pain, DIC, haemaglobinaemia and haemaglobinuria. Hypotension, not hypertension may also occur. Immediate haemolytic transfusion reactions are usually due to ABO incompatibility. Delayed haemolytic transfusion reactions may occur in patients alloimmunised by previous transfusions or pregnancies. The haemolysis is usually extravascular and the patient may develop anaemia and jaundice a week after transfusion (most are clinically silent).

47.   Colonoscopy   Answers: A D
Relative or absolute contraindications to colonoscopy include recent acute myocardial infarction, acute diverticulitis, acute moderate or severe colitis, peritonitis, and acute intestinal obstruction.

Classes of antibiotic

61.	Aztreonam	D	Monobactam
62.	Norfloxacin	B	Quinolone
63.	Erythromycin	A	Macrolide
64.	Vancomycin	C	Glycopeptide

Vancomycin is a glycopeptide antibiotic used for the treatment of resistant infections due to MRSA, *S. epidermidis* and *Cl. difficile*. It inhibits bacterial cell wall synthesis. Aztreonam contains a 5 monobactam ring and is resistant to β lactamase degradation. It is active against aerobic Gram negative organisms, and is an alternative to aminoglycosides.

Classification of organisms

65.	Cryptosporidium	B	Protozoal
66.	*Mycobacterium tuberculosis*	C	Bacterial
67.	*Pneumocystis carinii*	B	Protozoal
68.	*Cryptococcus neoformans*	A	Fungal
69.	Histoplasmosis	A	Fungal
70.	Aspergillus	A	Fungal
71.	*Nocardia asteroides*	A	Fungal
72.	*Listeria monocytogenes*	C	Bacterial

Immunosuppressed patients are prone to a variety of infective pathologies. These include fungal (histoplasmosis, aspergillosis, *Nocardia asteroides*, and *Cryptococcus neoformans*), protozoal (*Pneumocystis carinii* and cryptosporidiosis), bacterial (including *Mycobacterium tuberculosis* and *Listeria monocytogenes*), and viral organisms (measles virus, cytomegalovirus, Epstein-Barr virus, herpes simplex virus, and herpes zoster virus).

Arthropathy

73. B   Ankylosing spondylitis
74. A   Rheumatoid arthritis
75. H   Psoriatic arthritis
76. C   Reiter's syndrome

Rheumatoid arthritis is diagnosed on the basis of a bilateral symmetrical polyarthritis affecting the small joints of the hands and feet. Rheumatoid factor may be negative.

Ankylosing spondylitis and Reiter's syndrome are found mainly in young males. Rheumatoid factor is negative in both disorders. In ankylosing spondylitis, sacroiliac joint tenderness may be the only sign in the early stages as the classic stiffness of the spine does not appear until later in the disease. Males are affected more often than females.

Reiter's syndrome is a triad of arthritis, urethritis and conjunctivitis occurring some weeks after dysentery or sexually transmitted disease. Onset is usually between 20 and 40 years and males are affected ten times more commonly than females.

Psoriatic arthropathy is an erosive arthritis affecting typically the distal interphalangeal joints of the fingers. The rash of psoriasis may not be noted (especially if confined to the natal cleft or umbilicus), but nail pitting is common.

Calcium pyrophosphate disease or pseudogout typically presents as an acute asymmetrical large joint arthropathy. Calcium deposition in the cartilage of the knee is a characteristic feature.

Emergency resuscitation

77. E   Intravenous access (2 cannulae)
78. F   Chest drain insertion

In all cases where resuscitation is required, the airway must be addressed first, followed by the breathing along with administration of a high concentration of oxygen. Secure intravenous access is then required.

The first patient has evidence of circulatory failure (tachycardia, hypotension and poor peripheral perfusion). He requires urgent intravenous access followed by intravenous fluids.

The second patient has evidence of a massive haemothorax. Nevertheless, he is not oxygenating adequately despite a high FiO_2 and thus requires insertion of a chest drain immediately.

Chest trauma

79.	Restricted chest wall movement and rib crepitus	F Flail chest
80.	Shock associated with unilateral absent breath sounds and dullness to percussion	E Massive haemothorax
81.	Tracheal displacement to the opposite side	D Tension pneumothorax
82.	Muffled heart sounds and pulsus paradoxus	C Cardiac tamponade
83.	Pleural capping and tracheal deviation to the right	A Traumatic rupture of the thoracic aorta
84.	Depression of the left main bronchus and obliteration of the aorto-pulmonary window on CXR	A Traumatic rupture of the thoracic aorta

CXR findings of a traumatic rupture of the thoracic aorta (aortic dissection) include a widened mediastinum, pleural capping, oesophageal and tracheal deviation to the right, depression of the left main bronchus, and obliteration of the window between the pulmonary artery and aorta.

Massive haemothorax presents as shock associated with unilateral absence of breath sounds and dullness to percussion. Findings of a tension pneumothorax include tracheal displacement to the opposite side, respiratory distress, cyanosis, tachycardia, hypotension, distended neck veins, unilateral absent breath sounds and hyper-resonance. Cardiac tamponade is associated with muffled heart sounds, pulsus paradoxus and dilated neck veins. There is restricted chest wall movement with rib crepitus in cases of flail chest.

Testicular tumours

85.	Secretes alpha fetoprotein (αFP) in approximately 70% of cases	A Teratoma
86.	Secrete βhCG in less than 10% of cases	B Seminoma
87.	Secrete either αFP or βhCG in about 90% of cases	A Teratoma
88.	Secrete βhCG in approximately 60% of cases	A Teratoma
89.	Almost always secrete βhCG	C Choriocarcinoma

Teratomas produce αFP in about 70% of cases, secrete βhCG in about 60% of cases, and secrete either αFP or βhCG in about 90% of cases. Almost all choriocarcinomas secrete βhCG, but they do not produce αFP. Less than 10% of seminomas secrete βhCG, and very rarely produce αFP.

Chemotherapy regimens

90. Combination 5-fluorouracil and folinic acid   B   Colorectal carcinoma

91. Combination cyclophosphamide, methotrexate and 5-fluorouracil   D   Breast carcinoma

92. Combination bleomycin, cisplatin and etoposide   C   Testicular seminoma

Several studies have now shown limited survival benefit for Duke's C and Duke's B colorectal cancer using adjuvant treatment with combination 5-fluorouracil (5 FU) and folinic acid. Seminomas of the testis are sensitive to combination bleomycin, cisplatin and etoposide, and this has led to a marked improvement in survival in recent years. Adjuvant treatment for cancer of the breast using combination cyclophosphamide, methotrexate and 5 FU has been shown to prolong survival in premenopausal women who are node positive.

Peripheral nerve anatomy

93. C   Axillary
94. I   Thoracodorsal
95. G   Suprascapular
96. D   Radial
97. A   Long thoracic

• The axillary nerve passes just below the capsule of the shoulder joint and is damaged here in about 5% of shoulder dislocations. The nerve gives off the upper lateral cutaneous nerve of the arm, and also motor branches to the deltoid and teres minor muscles. The multipenate fibres of the deltoid muscle contract isometrically when carrying weights in the hand. The strap/unipenate anterior and posterior slips of the muscle are used for flexion and extension and, when contracting together, take over from the supraspinatus muscle to abduct the arm beyond the first 15º.

- The thoracodorsal nerve is most vulnerable to damage during axillary surgery, when the arm is laterally rotated and abducted, because it bows into the axilla from the posterior wall. Paralysis of the latissimus dorsi muscle is detected clinically if the patient is unable to fold the arm behind the back and reach up to the opposite scapula.

- The suprascapular nerve, which is motor to the supraspinatus and infraspinatus muscles, may be damaged by sudden tightening of a car seat belt (upper trunk injuries of the brachial plexus and clavicular fractures may also occur). Paralysis of both muscles weakens the rotator cuff, destabilising the shoulder joint. In addition, supraspinatus abducts the arm over the first 15°, and infraspinatus is a powerful lateral rotator of the humerus. Since the teres minor muscle is unaffected (axillary nerve), some lateral rotation is preserved after suprascapular nerve damage.

- Mid shaft fractures of the humerus can damage the radial nerve in the spiral groove. The branches to the triceps are given off before the nerve enters the groove and so the muscle remains functional. All other extensors are paralysed so resulting in wrist drop. Although the cutaneous branches no longer conduct, compensatory overlap by adjacent nerves restricts the paraesthesia/anaesthesia to the dorsal skin over the first interosseous muscle. The brachioradialis reflex is mediated by the radial nerve and is thus lost. The triceps reflex remains intact for reasons explained above.

- The long thoracic nerve usually escapes damage during axillary surgery because it is bound to the serratus anterior muscle by overlying fascia on the medial wall, posterior to the mid axillary line. When the nerve is injured, however, part or all of the serratus anterior muscle is paralysed, resulting in a 'winged scapula'. There is loss of protraction and weakness of rotation of the scapula (the later movement is however preserved by the action of the intact trapezius muscle - spinal accessory nerve).

Anatomy of lungs and airways   Answers:

98. Is separated from the arch of the aorta by the vagus nerve   D   Left pulmonary artery
99. Lies behind the left brachiocephalic vein   F   Trachea
100. Is the most anterior structure in the hilum   E   Left pulmonary vein
101. Lies anterior to the oesophagus   G   Lobes of the lungs
102. Bifurcates outside the lung   A   Left main bronchus

- The left pulmonary artery is separated from the arch of the aorta by the left vagus, the recurrent laryngeal nerve, and the ligamentum arteriosum.
- The left brachiocephalic vein passes in front of the trachea in the midline.
- The left upper pulmonary vein is the most anterior structure in the left hilum.
- There are 10 bronchopulmonary segments in each lung despite the left middle lobe being diminutive; 3 in the upper, 2 in the middle, and 5 in the lower lobes.
- The left main bronchus is longer than the right and crosses in front of the oesophagus, providing a potential obstruction to food during deglutition.

Brachial plexus and nerves of upper arm

103.A   C5, C6, C7 roots of brachial plexus
104.B   C8, T1 roots of brachial plexus
105.C   Long thoracic nerve
106.E   Axillary nerve
107.F   Radial nerve

Erb's palsy (upper brachial plexus injury) may be found after difficult deliveries. It is much more common than Klumpke's paralysis (the corresponding lower brachial plexus injury).

Pure lower brachial plexus injuries are rare. The presence of Horner's syndrome suggests C8 and T1 root avulsion and helps to differentiate this injury from an ulnar nerve lesion. It is essential to establish how proximal the injury is in these cases as pre-ganglionic avulsions are irreparable whereas post-ganglionic avulsions may be amenable to repair.

Injuries of the long thoracic nerve (of Bell) may occur following axillary dissection. Damage to the axillary nerve may occur after shoulder dislocation.

In addition to loss of deltoid contraction, there may be loss of sensation in the badge area although this is not universal. Recovery usually occurs within three months, but on occasions the nerve is completely divided and requires repair or shoulder stabilization.

'Saturday night palsy' of the radial nerve is not uncommon after drinking binges. The usual mechanism is direct pressure on the nerve in the spiral groove of the humerus as the arm hangs over the back of a chair. Recovery is usual.

Peripheral nerves of the upper limb

108.G Deep branch of ulnar nerve
109.E Anterior interosseous nerve
110.C Ulnar nerve

The ulnar nerve divides into its deep (motor) and superficial (sensory) branches as it leaves the canal of Guyon. The deep branch is prone to compression where it passes round the pisiform bone in the palm.

The anterior interosseous branch of the median nerve (which supplies the flexor pollicis longus and flexor digitorum profundus to the index and middle fingers) may be compressed (usually by muscle hypertrophy from repeated forced pronation) where it passes through pronator teres, giving rise to muscle weakness but no motor signs.

One of the commonest nerve compressions is of the ulnar nerve at the cubital tunnel. Although the nerve is a mixed nerve, sensory signs and symptoms predominate in the early stages as the smaller diameter of the sensory fibres renders them more prone to neuropraxia

Acquired coagulation disorders

111.PT	28	APTT	56	TT 22	FIB	2.5	B	Established warfarin therapy
112.PT	14	APTT	58	TT 11	FIB	3.1	E	Acquired von Willebrand's disease
113.PT	16	APTT	52	TT 124	FIB	1.9	A	Heparin therapy
114.PT	15	APTT	37	TT 12	FIB	2.9	C	Aspirin therapy
115.PT	24	APTT	49	TT 28	FIB	0.9	D	Hepatic insufficiency

Prolongation of all the clotting times and reduced fibrinogen implies a global factor synthetic defect which can only be explained by hepatic insufficiency. Warfarin also prolongs the PT but after 1–2 days of treatment, its action on the synthesis of Factors II, IX and X leads to prolongation of the APTT and TT. Both heparin and acquired von Willebrand's disease cause prolongation of the APPT with preservation of the PT, but heparin also inhibits the polymerisation of fibrin and so prolongs the TT. Isolated defects in platelet function such as in aspirin therapy may produce significant bleeding yet have a normal coagulation screen and full blood count. Abnormalities in specific platelet aggregation assays are seen.

Diagnosis of acute blood transfusion reactions

116. C   Anaphylactic reaction
117. F   Acute haemolytic transfusion reaction
118. A   Non-haemolytic febrile transfusion reaction

Acute circulatory collapse shortly after starting transfusion may occur in acute haemolytic transfusion reactions or transfusion of contaminated blood products. However, wheezing, tachypnoea and tachycardia are more typical of anaphylaxis which is usually due to a brisk primary immune response to a plasma protein. Acute haemolysis is very unusual in fresh frozen plasma transfusion and since plasma is frozen shortly after separation it is unlikely that bacterial contaminants would have time to replicate to sufficient levels to produce overt septic shock. Haemolytic transfusion reactions to non-ABO antigens are characteristically less severe than ABO incompatible reactions. The presentation described in scenario 2 is classical of haemolysis due to non-ABO antigens and results from red cell destruction in the reticulo-endothelial system. Delayed haemolytic transfusion reactions are secondary antibody reactions that lead to extra-vascular haemolysis usually 10–15 days after transfusion. Milder transfusion reactions are common and usually present with malaise, headache, nausea usually with a mild pyrexia. The lack of itching or a skin rash and the rapid response to paracetamol described in scenario 3 suggests a non-haemolytic febrile transfusion reaction. This is usually caused by a primary immune response against previously encountered white cell antigen and is most common in parous women and recipients of previous transfusions.

END OF CORE PAPER 4

1.   Circulating blood volume   Answers: A B D F

Vasoconstriction is widespread and occurs on both the venous and arterial sides of the circulation. The result is increased peripheral resistance to blood flow. Changes in vascular pressures lead to an influx of extracellular water into the circulation, a phenomenon known as transcapillary refilling. This leads to haemodilution. Tachycardia occurs as a fall in blood pressure is sensed by baroreceptors in the carotid arteries and aortic arch.

2.   Central venous line   Answers: All true

Central venous line insertion may cause trauma to adjacent tissues with consequent haemorrhage and pneumothorax. If it is left open then air may enter the blood causing venous air embolism. Systemic arterial air embolism may occur if the cannula is mistakenly placed in the carotid artery.

3.   Wound infection   Answers: A C E

General host factors predisposing to wound infection include hypoxia, jaundice, anaemia, increasing age, obesity, uraemia, malnutrition, diabetes mellitus, hypovolaemic shock, corticosteroids, and immuno-suppressants.

4.   Cardiopulmonary bypass   Answer: B

Cardiopulmonary bypass is often associated with thrombocytopenia and platelet dysfunction. It is usually combined with induced hypothermia to reduce tissue metabolic demand. Plasma coagulation factor levels drop due to haemodilution. Heparin is routinely used to prevent extracorporeal clotting in the oxygenator. Protamine sulphate is used at the end of bypass to neutralise remaining circulating heparin.

5.   ARDS   Answers: A C E

Physiological and histological features of ARDS include increased capillary permeability, interstitial and alveolar oedema, fibrin exudation, hyaline membrane formation, and diffuse late interstitial and alveolar fibrosis.

6.   **Respiratory failure**   **Answers: A E**

In acute respiratory failure the PaO_2 falls and the $PaCO_2$ rises with a consequent drop in pH. In chronic respiratory failure, the serum bicarbonate increases to correct acidaemia. The increase of bicarbonate in the CSF renders the respiratory centre in the brainstem insensitive to hypercarbia but not hypoxia. Thus a hypoxic respiratory drive takes over and is the only stimulus to increase ventilation rate.

7.   **Central venous pressure**   **Answer: B**

The CVP reflects pressure in the right atrium and would thus be elevated in right-sided heart failure. The CVP is low in all types of shock except for cardiogenic shock. CVP does not directly reflect cardiac output but at best is merely an indicator of intravascular fluid volume.

8.   **Acute renal failure**   **Answers: B C D**

Acute renal failure (ARF) occurs in about 30% critically ill patients. Loss of renal function leads to a 60% increase in mortality and morbidity. The common causes of ARF include post-operative hypovolaemia, CCF, radio-contrast and drugs (aminoglycosides, NSAIDs). 20% of ARF is drug induced. In 60% cases, ARF is potentially avoidable, as it is the result of fluid or drug mismanagement. The histological appearance of the kidney bears little relevance to the level of renal dysfunction. Minimal damage can result in fairly severe functional deficit. The proximal tubule is the segment that is most susceptible to injury and reflects the relative hypoxia in the outer medulla and inner cortex.

9.   **Penetrating hepatic trauma**   **Answers: A B E**

Penetrating hepatic trauma in the unstable patient requires emergency treatment but can, occasionally, in stable patients, be managed conservatively. It usually presents with hypotension and shock but can sometimes present late with symptoms such as haemobilia. It is rarely fatal if treated aggressively. At operation, excessive bleeding is usually controlled by pressure, direct suture or packing swabs around the liver but not into the hepatic defect. Pringle's manoeuvre consists of intermittent compression of the free edge of the lesser omentum (contains the portal vein and hepatic artery) to staunch the haemorrhage.

10. 'Open' or 'sucking' pneumothorax   Answers: A B E

Air passes preferentially through the chest wall with each respiratory effort along the path of least resistance, reducing alveolar ventilation and resulting in tissue hypoxia. Sealing the chest wall defect completely may result in a tension pneumothorax. Acute treatment is by creation of a flap valve dressing to occlude the defect during inspiration but allowing expulsion of intra-pleural air during exhalation. A chest drain can later be placed at a site away from the chest wall defect. Defects themselves usually require definitive surgical closure.

11. Flail chest   Answers: A C D

Flail chest occurs when a chest wall segment loses bony continuity with the rest of the thoracic cage, usually resulting from trauma associated with multiple rib fractures. Disruption of the normal chest wall movement and underlying lung contusion may cause the major problems resulting in hypoxia. Diagnosis may be difficult because of splinting of the chest wall. Treatment includes oxygen therapy with establishment of adequate ventilation (frequently requires artificial ventilation), management of associated lung contusion by carefully controlling fluid infusions. However, it does not take priority over aggressive fluid management if the patient is hypotensive.

12. Acute cervical spine injuries   Answers: B E

Good quality lateral cervical spine films will pick up approximately 90% of significant cervical spine injuries in adults. An acceptable quality lateral cervical spine X-ray should include the upper border of T1 so as to exclude a cervico-thoracic dislocation.

Significant cervical spine injury may be found even in the absence of radiological abnormalities on standard views, particularly in children. Spinal cord injury without radiological abnormality is commoner in children than in adults.

13. Acute extradural haematoma   Answers: C D

Extradural haematomas are usually biconvex in appearance. In contrast to subdural haematomas, they may be seen to cross the midline, but do not usually cross suture lines. Decreased attenuation of a haematoma is usually a feature of a chronic (over 21 days old) subdural haematoma.

14.   Major incidence planning   Answers: A B C
Major incidence planning requires involvement of senior police, fire and ambulance officials. Response plans should be formally recorded and intermittently tested. Adequate communication facilities are essential to co-ordinate tactical response. Patients already hospitalised for conditions unrelated to the disaster should not be routinely evacuated but provisions made for their immediate urgent needs. Disaster co-ordination should be by the most senior hospital staff - consultants and administrators.

15.   Acute compartment syndrome   Answers: B D
Compartment syndrome usually presents with excessive pain despite limb immobilisation. The patient will usually have pain on passive movement (later feature) and often has distal paraesthesia. Loss of distal pulses and distal pallor are late features and do not usually occur until after irreversible muscle necrosis supervenes.

16.   Multi-trauma patient   Answers: A E
A minimum of two large gauge venflons (14G) in the ante-cubital fossae should be established during the early assessment of severely traumatised patients. ATLS recommends that initial fluid replacement should be with a balanced salt solution (Ringer's lactate solution). Hypovolaemic shock is treated with intravenous volume replacement. Vasopressive agents have no role in the initial stage.

17.   Medications   Answers: A C E
Stopping anti-hypertensive medication prior to surgery may lead to significant intra-operative swings in blood pressure. Therefore, they should be continued. Mono amine oxidase increases the bio-availability of catecholamines. Thus, cessation of MAOIs may lead to extreme hypertension during surgery so increasing the risk of cardiac and neurological complications.

18.   Malignant melanoma   Answers: A B C D
Clinical stage of disease is the single most important prognostic factor, followed by the thickness of the primary tumour (Breslow's thickness), as measured from the granular cell layer of the epidermis to the deepest easily identifiable tumour cell. Other prognostic factors include sex (females have a better prognosis), ulceration (worse prognosis), age (< 50 years do better) and the site: the limbs have a better prognosis than the trunk, which has a better prognosis than the head and neck. The degree of melanosis is not a prognostic factor.

19.   Malignant potential   Answers: A B

Solar keratosis has a malignant potential but is not a carcinoma *in situ*. Keratoacanthoma is a benign self-involuting lesion, and molluscum contagiosum is an infective lesion. Basal cell papillomas (seborrhoeic keratosis) are benign and have no malignant potential.

20.   Cutaneous squamous cell carcinomas   Answers: A B D F

Xeroderma pigmentosa is an autosomal recessive disorder in which there is increased susceptibility to sunlight-induced skin damage. There is a >1000 times increased risk of developing cutaneous SCCs in xeroderma pigmentosa. SCCs never regress to produce Bowen's disease. A SCC seen in a long-standing venous ulcer is known as a Marjolin's ulcer. There is an increased incidence of cutaneous SCC in renal transplant recipients, and other chronically immunocompromised patients. Less than 5% of cutaneous SCCs metastasise to lymph nodes. SCCs on the vulva and penis behave in a more aggressive fashion and thus have a worse prognosis. A Spitz naevus is a variant of benign melanocytic lesions and can be mistaken histologically for malignant melanoma. They are more common in females < 30 years.

21.   Malignant tumours   Answers: A B D E

Staging of malignant lesions for individual patients allows only a statistical risk of outcome for that patient. Accurate tumour staging cannot be made on the basis of a histological specimen alone, and requires additional information on nodal and distant disease. Pathological staging may be altered by response to chemotherapy or irradiation treatment, and is known as 'downstaging'. Staging of tumours takes into account local tissue anatomy for individual primary tumour sites e.g. invasion of tumours into the different layers of the wall of any viscus, and invasion into adjacent local structures.

22.   Colorectal carcinoma   Answers: B C D

The vast majority of colorectal carcinomas are thought to arise from pre-existing polyps. There is an increased incidence of development of colorectal carcinoma following ureterosigmoidostomy, especially in the vicinity of the anastomosis. Chromosome 17 and 18 abnormalities are common and are thought to be involved in the progression of adenomatous polyps to carcinoma. Duke's A tumours are confined to the muscularis propria, Duke's B tumours are confined to the bowel wall, and Duke's C tumours have lymph node involvement. Longitudinal tumour spread is not a marked feature of colorectal carcinoma, and distal intramural spread > 1 cm beyond the gross margins of the tumour is uncommon.

23.   Malignant testicular tumours   Answers: A B F

Testicular tumours account for < 1% of all male tumours, but their incidence is rising. Germ-cell tumours (teratomas (35%), seminomas (50%), and mixed seminoma-teratomas (15%)), account for almost 90% of all malignant testicular neoplasms. Seminomas are more radiosensitive than teratomas. Teratomas have a greater metastatic potential and a worse prognosis than seminomas.

24.   Screening for breast cancer   Answers: A B

Mammographic screening for early breast cancers has been shown to reduce deaths from breast cancer by up to 30%, and to reduce the incidence of Stage II disease by 25%. The incidence of detecting breast cancer in screened patients aged 50–64 years is 4 per 1000 at prevalence screening, and 1 per 1000 at subsequent screening. The ideal frequency of further examinations is debated but presently occurs every three years. The incidence of breast cancer in patients aged under 40 years is too low to justify its use.

25.   Phylloides tumours   Answers: B C E

Approximately 20% of phylloides tumours of the breast are malignant. These tumours have a benign epithelial component, and a stromal component which can be either benign or malignant. These tumours are frequently large, and on cut section are fleshy and lobulated. Malignant lesions spread via bloodstream, and regional nodal spread is rare.

26.   Adjuvant chemotherapy   Answers: B C

Drugs given in combination appear to give better results than drugs in isolation. The most popular present combination is cyclophosphamide, methotrexate and 5 fluorouracil (CMF). The drugs are most commonly given by intermittent injection although there is increasing interest in continuous infusion via intra-arterial or intravenous pumps. Chemotherapy is the treatment of choice for visceral metastases (especially liver and brain), and for inflammatory cancers. The clinical response is not only confined to pre-menopausal women, though the gain in survival is approximately 5%.

27. Pre-malignant conditions   Answers: A C E

Balanitis xerotica obliterans is a dyskeratotic skin disorder affecting the prepuce, glans or urethral meatus. There is no associated malignancy. Paget's disease of the breast is associated with underlying breast malignancy and, therefore, is not a pre-malignant condition. Both Peutz-Jeghers syndrome and familial adenomatous polyposis predispose to malignancies in the small bowel (2% risk) and large bowel (100% risk by 30 years) respectively. Severe dysplasia in a Barrett's oesophagus may also progress to oesophageal adenocarcinoma, the risk being approximately twenty-fold.

28. Breast cysts   Answers: B D

Aspiration of breast cysts usually reveals clear or brownish fluid. Cysts returning blood-stained fluid should be biopsied, as it may reflect an associated intraductal carcinoma. If cysts are simple, there should be no residual lump following aspiration. Residual lumps and recurrent cysts should be biopsied to exclude underlying malignancy. If cysts are simple, 90% will not recur following aspiration.

29. Split skin grafting   Answers: B D

In optimal conditions for SSG there should be no bacterial growth from the wound. However, split skin grafting is usually successful in the presence of most skin commensals including *Staphylococcus epidermidis*, *Staphylococcus aureus* (including MRSA) and Klebsiella. *Beta-haemolytic streptococci* and Pseudomonas both produce toxins which prevent split skin grafts from 'taking'.

30. Viral hepatitis   Answers: A D

Hepatitis A is an RNA virus and hepatitis B a DNA virus. The incubation period of hepatitis A is between 2–3 weeks. Hepatitis A accounts for 20–40% of all cases of viral hepatitis. It affects children and young adults particularly. It rarely causes fulminant hepatitis and does not give rise to a carrier state.

31. Post-splenectomy sepsis   Answers: A E

The risk of post-splenectomy sepsis is reduced by pneumococcal and HiB (*Haemophilus influenzae*) vaccination, as well as by maintenance prophylactic oral antibiotics (penicillin or amoxycillin). The vaccinations should be administered at least two weeks before splenectomy. The meningococcal vaccine is presently only recommended for those patients travelling to endemic areas or those who are immunocompromised.

32.   Diathermy   Answers: B C
Diathermy uses the heating effect of electrical current. The smaller area
the current travels through the higher the current density and the greater
the heating effect. A high frequency current is used as this causes fewer
problems e.g. unpleasant sensations, muscle contraction and ventricular
fibrillation. However, high frequency electricity can spark across gaps
and a patient may receive an exit burn even though he is not touching
an earth. Class 3 equipment is incapable of producing a burn. Diathermy
can be used in a patient with a pacemaker but the pad of a monopolar
diathermy should be positioned well away from the pacemaker. Bipolar
diathermy does not interfere with pacemakers and may be more suitable.

33.   Spinal hemi-section   Answer: D
Unilateral C5/6 cord lesions are at the lower level of origin of the
phrenic nerve (C3, 4, 5, mainly C4) so respiration is unaffected. Shoulder
shrugging is mediated by the spinal accessory nerve (C1–C4), and
cutaneous sensation over the clavicle (C4 dermatome) is mediated by
the supraclavicular nerves. Spinal lesions lead to ipsilateral loss of fine
touch and contralateral loss of pain and temperature sensation below the
lesion.

34.   Transthoracic plane of Louis   Answer: A
Structures within the transthoracic plane (of Louis) include the azygos
vein and left recurrent laryngeal nerve looping round the ligamentum
arteriosum. The bifurcation of the pulmonary trunk lies below and the
upper border of the aortic arch above the plane.

35.   Bronchial metastases   Answers: B C E
Hilar metastases could damage the phrenic nerve anteriorly, the vagus
posteriorly, and left recurrent laryngeal nerve superiorly. Phrenic nerve
damage could cause paralysis of the ipsilateral diaphragm, which would
be raised on a PA chest X-ray,and could cause paraesthesia referred to
the C4 dermatome. Laryngeal stridor and dyspnoea would follow
destruction of the left recurrent laryngeal nerve. Obstruction of the left
main bronchus by enlarged nodes may also contribute to the dyspnoea.
Spread would occur over the left tracheobronchial nodes and would not
usually involve the infraclavicular nodes.

36.   L5 nerve root compression   Answers: A C D
The commonest cause of L5 root compression is a prolapsed
intervertebral disc. Signs include weakness of the extensor hallucis
longus, weakness of ankle dorsiflexion, wasting of extensor digitorum
brevis, and reduced sensation in the L5 dermatome.

37. The right atrium   Answers: A B C D

The right atrium forms the right border of the heart, lies anterior to the left atrium and thus the posterior wall is the inter-atrial septum. The sinoatrial node lies near the opening of the superior vena cava, lateral to the sulcus limitans, and the coronary sinus opens into the atrium above both the opening of the inferior vena cava, and septal cusp of the tricuspid valve.

38. Acute haemolytic transfusion reaction   Answers: C E

The intravenous giving set should be removed but the cannula retained as iv access is required. The patient should be given large quantities of iv fluids in order to promote a urine output of > 1.5 ml/kg/hr. Frusemide should be given to promote diuresis and if the patient remains oliguric a central line should be inserted. 100 ml of 20% mannitol is recommended for 'renal protection'. Hyperkalaemia and DIC may both occur and require specific treatment.

39. Prothrombin time   Answers: A D E

The prothrombin time measures the integrity of the extrinsic and common pathways of coagulation and is therefore sensitive to deficiency or inhibition of factors II, V, VII and X. It is particularly sensitive to the global impairment of coagulation factor synthesis seen in severe liver disease or to vitamin K deficiency (impaired synthesis of factors II, VII, IX and X). Coagulation factor deficiencies, which affect only the intrinsic pathway such as haemophilia A (Factor VIII deficiency), will not prolong the prothrombin time. The prothrombin time is usually expressed as an international normalised ratio (INR) when monitoring oral anticoagulant dose. This allows standardisation of reagents between different laboratories.

40. Intravascular haemolysis   Answers: B D E

Intravascular haemolysis may result from the mechanical destruction of red cells by prosthetic heart valves or arterial grafts, in arterio-venous malformations or after severe physical exercise. Immune mediated intravascular haemolysis is only usually encountered in the potent antibody-antigen interactions that are seen following ABO mismatched transfusion. Most auto-immune haemolytic anaemias produce red cell destruction in the reticulo-endothelial system. Disseminated intra-vascular coagulation may cause microangiopathic haemolysis with red cell destruction in the microcirculation.

41.   Anticoagulant therapy

Answers: A B D E

Bleeding is the most frequent complication of both warfarin and heparin therapy although there is now evidence that the incidence is lower with low molecular weight heparins than unfractionated heparin. Warfarin is teratogenic in high doses and in most cases should be avoided in pregnancy. Idiosyncratic reactions to warfarin include skin necrosis, skin reactions, hepatic dysfunction and pancreatitis. Heparin induced thrombocytopenia is an immune mediated disorder that usually develops after 6–10 days of treatment and paradoxically is associated with thrombosis. Platelet counts should be monitored in individuals receiving heparin for longer than five days. In the event of a falling platelet count, heparin should be discontinued and an alternative anticoagulant instituted. Other side-effects of heparin include osteoporosis, skin necrosis and hypersensitivity reactions.

42.   Platelet count

Answers: B D E

Thrombocytopenia is a common haematological abnormality and usually arises from increased peripheral destruction of platelets in disorders such as immune thrombocytopenia, disseminated intravascular coagulation, hypersplenism or following heparin therapy. Thrombocytopenia may also occur in infiltrative bone marrow disorders such as carcinomatosis. Artefactual thrombocytopenia may result from platelet clumping *in vitro* following difficult venesection. Spontaneous bleeding in an afebrile patient, with otherwise normal haemostasis is unlikely at platelet counts greater than $10 \times 10^9/l$. Thrombocytosis may indicate an acute phase response in sepsis, inflammatory disorders or malignancy. It is common for the platelet count to rise transiently after splenectomy.

43.   Autologous blood transfusion

Answer: C

Autologous blood transfusion involves the collection and storage of the patient's own blood in advance of an elective surgical procedure. Since red cell donations have a shelf life of 35 days, it is usually only possible to collect 2–4 units pre-operatively. Blood must be ABO and rhesus D tested and compatibility tested, labelled and stored to the same standard as donor blood. This technique has theoretical advantages in that it reduces the risk of serological reactions and transmission of some infectious agents. There is still, however, the risk of clerical error and bacterial contamination. Not all patients are fit enough to tolerate pre-operative blood donation and some patients will need additional transfusion of donor units after unforeseen bleeding. Autologous transfusion is unacceptable to Jehovah's Witness patients.

44.   Massive blood transfusion   Answers: A B C D

Massive blood transfusion is defined as replacement of the whole blood volume within 24 hours. Since red cell donations contain few platelets and low concentrations of coagulation factors, dilutional thrombocytopenia and coagulopathy can occur. Other sequelae include: hypocalcaemia, hyperkalaemia and metabolic alkalosis. Correction of these biochemical and haematological abnormalities should be on an 'as needed' basis. Hypothermia is a recognised hazard and a blood warmer should be used routinely. Adult respiratory distress syndrome is a well recognised complication.

45.   Cryoprecipitates   Answers: C D

Cryoprecipitates are concentrates which include factor VIII, fibrinogen and von Willebrand factor. Platelets, factor VI and fresh frozen plasma are not components. Cryoprecipitate may be used for haemophilia, von Willebrand's disease and disseminated intravascular coagulation. However, factor specific cryoprecipitates are becoming more readily available.

46.   Iron deficiency anaemia   Answers: B D

Iron deficiency anaemia is associated with the symptoms and signs of anaemia: brittle spoon shaped nails (koilonychia), glossitis, angular cheilitis, developmental delay in children and, rarely, dysphagia from a crico-pharyngeal web (Plummer-Vinson or Paterson-Kelly-Brown syndrome). Occasionally pica for materials such as ice and clay occurs. Neurological abnormalities are the hallmark of B_{12} deficiency. Laboratory investigations in iron deficiency anaemia show a microcytic, hypochromic picture, a characteristic blood film, reduced serum ferritin, increased serum iron binding capacity and reduced transferrin saturation.

47.   Clinical trials   Answers: A C

Single blinding refers to the patient not knowing which treatment he/she has received. Double blinding is when both the patient and the investigator are unaware which treatment the patient is receiving. A control group is a group of patients observed after not receiving the index treatment. Historical controls are not as reliable as a group randomised to control.

SECTION 2 – EMQs

Cardiorespiratory arrest

61. G
62. A
63. D
64. H
65. I
66. B

Resuscitation always addresses and corrects the airway first, then the breathing, followed by circulation. The published European Resuscitation Council (ERC) guidelines provide an essential framework for the management of cardiac arrest and also for peri-arrest dysrhythmias. Surgery may be part of the resuscitation, as in the patient with the ante-partum haemorrhage. There are didactic protocols by the ERC which vary depending on the rhythm. These should be followed when managing a cardiac arrest. The precordial thump is part of ALS practice, but is only advised when a patient in VF has a witnessed cardiac arrest.

Investigations for DVT

67. Indicates the extent and degree of fixity of thrombus   D   Phlebography
68. Is contraindicated in the presence of severe peripheral vascular disease   D   Phlebography
69. Has a 50% false-positive rate   A   Clinical examination
70. Lower limb incisions can give false-positives   E   Radioiodine-labelled fibrinogen scan
71. Has a risk of inducing hepatitis   E   Radioiodine-labelled fibrinogen scan

Clinical examination is notoriously inaccurate for the identification of DVT, with a 50% false-negative and false-positive rate. Doppler ultrasound (duplex) is now the most widely used method of assessment, and is extremely reliable for thrombus at or above the popliteal fossa. Impedance plethysmography is not widely used, but may be best used to detect major vein thrombosis. Phlebography will usually be able to demonstrate the extent and degree of fixity of the thrombus. However, it is contraindicated in severe peripheral vascular disease. Radioiodine-labelled fibrinogen scans do not give accurate results above mid thigh level. They are associated with false-positives after lower limb incisions, contraindicated during pregnancy and may induce hepatitis. It tends to be used primarily as a research tool.

Benign lesions of skin and lymphatics

72. Lymphatic channels   D   Cystic hygroma
73. Apocrine gland   B   Cylindroma
74. Synovial sheath   C   Ganglion
75. Eccrine gland   E   Syringoma
76. Hair follicle   A   Pilomatrixoma

A pilomatrixoma is a common subcutaneous, often calcified, nodule of hair follicle origin. It occurs mostly on the face or scalp of young adults. A cylindroma (apocrine gland origin) typically occurs on the scalp and may be multiple. When extensive it may cover the scalp and is then known as a 'turban tumour'. A ganglion is a cystic degeneration of a synovial tendon sheath. A cystic hygroma is a lymphangioma resulting from failure of local lymphatics to communicate with the main lymphatic system. Syringomas are small cutaneous nodules of eccrine gland origin occurring mostly on the eyelids, neck, chest and genitalia of young adults. They may be multiple.

Mode of tumour spread

77. Seminoma of the testis	D	Lymphatic spread
78. Cutaneous basal cell carcinoma	A	Local invasion
79. Papillary thyroid carcinoma	D	Lymphatic spread
80. Follicular thyroid carcinoma	B	Blood-borne spread
81. Ovarian carcinoma	C	Transcoelomic spread

Seminomas of the testis and papillary thyroid carcinoma are spread predominantly by the lymphatic route. Cutaneous basal cell carcinomas invade local structures after many years of neglect. They rarely, if ever, spread to lymphatics or metastasise. Follicular thyroid carcinomas are spread predominantly by the bloodstream. Ovarian carcinomas frequently spread transcoelomically.

Thyroid cancer

82. Early haematogenous and lymphatic spread	D	Anaplastic carcinoma
83. Is usually very radiosensitive	E	Lymphoma
84. Accounts for 60% of thyroid carcinoma cases	A	Papillary carcinoma
85. Is derived from parafollicular C cells	C	Medullary cell carcinoma
86. Commonly metastasises to bone and lung but lymphatic spread is unusual	B	Follicular carcinoma

Papillary carcinoma of the thyroid are 4 times more common in women. They tend to exhibit multicentricity and metastasize to lymph nodes early. Follicular carcinoma of the thyroid, in contrast, tends to be solitary, encapsulated, invades the bloodstream and spreads to bone.
Medullary thyroid cancer is sporadic in 90% of cases. Familial cases may be associated with MEN II. Calcitonin a good tumour marker for medullary thyroid cancer. Anaplastic carcinoma has one of the worst prognoses. It is a very aggressive tumour invading all local structures early.

Bone and joint sepsis

87. F β-haemolytic streptococcus
88. B *Staphylococcus aureus*
89. A *Mycobacterium tuberculosis*
90. C *Haemophilus influenzae*
91. G *Clostridium perfringens*

A spreading cellulitis is classically associated with a Streptococcal infection. Whilst a child with sickle cell disease is at risk of developing an osteomyelitis with *Salmonella typhi*, the most common organism is still *Staphylococcus aureus*. Even if the X-ray features do not suggest osteomyelitis the diagnosis must be considered until it can be excluded. One must consider TB as the cause of a chronic infection in an immunosuppressed patient with sinus formation. The cause of septic arthritis varies with the age of the child – in a toddler, particularly one recovering from a URTI, *H. Influenzae* is the most likely organism. In an injury with a dirty wound and systematic features – gas gangrene needs to be considered with *Clostridium perfringens* as the causative organism.

Trauma

92. E Ruptured diaphragm
93. C Basal skull fracture
94. A Flail chest
95. G Jefferson's fracture
96. D Fractured 1st rib
97. B Fracture of C3

Trauma resuscitation follows the ABC principles of ATLS training. In multiple trauma, the initial assessment will include three X-rays (chest, cervical spine and pelvis) which are likely to yield most information of clinical significance during the resuscitative stage of management. If there is no neck tenderness and no focal neurology, a cervical spine X-ray may not be indicated. A full secondary survey is necessary to identify other less serious injuries, and also to detect deterioration or the development of new pathology. Battle's sign may not become obvious until several hours after injury.

Pelvic fracture

98. Lateral compression fracture   B   Rotationally unstable, vertically stable pelvic fracture
99. Open book fracture   B   Rotationally unstable, vertically stable pelvic fracture
100. Vertical shear injuries   C   Rotationally unstable, vertically unstable pelvic fracture
101. Isolated iliac wing fracture   A   Stable pelvic fracture
102. Isolated pubic ramus fracture   A   Stable pelvic fracture

Stable pelvic fractures include fractures not displacing the pelvic ring, such as avulsion fractures and isolated fractures of the iliac wing or pubic ramus, or minimally displaced fractures of the pelvic ring. Rotationally unstable, vertically stable pelvic fractures include open book fractures (pubic diastasis > 2.5 cm) and lateral compression fractures. Rotationally and vertically unstable pelvic fractures usually result from vertical shear injuries.

Burns

103. Burns to all the head and neck	D	9%
104. Burns to all the anterior trunk (chest/abdomen)	F	18%
105. Burns to all the male genitals	A	1%
106. Burns to all the posterior trunk (upper and lower back)	F	18%
107. Burns to the whole anterior aspect of one leg	D	9%
108. Burns to the whole anterior aspect of one arm	B	4.5%
109. Burns to the whole posterior aspect of both legs	F	18%

The rule of nines gives a practical guide to the rapid calculation of the extent of body burns. The adult body is divided into anatomical regions comprising 9% of the total body surface. The head and neck comprise 9% of the total body surface, the anterior trunk (chest and abdomen) 18%, the posterior chest (upper and lower) 18%, each arm 9%, and each leg 18%. The genitals comprise 1% of total body surface area.

Multiple Endocrine Neoplasia

110. Submucosal neuromas   C   Multiple Endocrine Neoplasia IIB
111. Pancreatic islet cell   A   Multiple Endocrine Neoplasia I
    adenomas
112. Marfanoid appearance   C   Multiple Endocrine Neoplasia IIB
113. Pituitary hyperplasia   A   Multiple Endocrine Neoplasia I

The Multiple Endocrine Neoplasia syndromes are inherited in an autosomal dominant manner or occur as new mutations. MEN I consists of pituitary, pancreatic islet cell and parathyroid adenomas or hyperplasia. Patients with MEN IIA and IIB develop phaeochromocytomas and medullary thyroid carcinomas. In addition, those with MEN IIA develop parathyroid hyperplasia, but are phenotypically normal, but those with MEN IIB tend to be Marfanoid and develop submucosal neuromas.

Anatomy of brachial plexus

114. Is formed by branches from   G   Median nerve
    two different cords
115. Gives off the suprascapular nerve   C   Upper trunk
116. Has no contribution from   B   Posterior cord
    anterior divisions
117. Is formed from a single anterior   F   Medial cord
    division
118. Is a direct continuation of the   D   Middle trunk
    C7 root
119. Innervates the entire flexor   H   Anterior divisions
    compartment of the upper limb
120. Receives a grey ramus from the   A   C7 root
    inferior cervical (or stellate)
    sympathetic ganglion
121. Contributes a branch to the   E   C6 root
    long thoracic nerve (of Bell)

- The median nerve is formed from medial and lateral heads of the medial and lateral cords, respectively.
- Only the upper trunk of the plexus possesses a branch, the suprascapular nerve.
- The posterior cord is formed entirely by posterior divisions.
- The medial cord is a continuation of the anterior division of the medial trunk; there is no other contribution to the medial cord.

- The middle trunk is a direct continuation of the C7 root; there is no other contribution to the middle trunk.
- Anterior divisions innervate the flexor compartment of the limbs.
- The inferior cervical sympathetic ganglion sends post-ganglionic fibres to the C7 and C8 roots - other sympathetic contributions to the plexus are from the T1 ganglion to the T1 root, and the middle cervical ganglion to the C5 and C6 roots (the superior ganglion contributes grey rami to the upper 4 cervical nerves).
- The long thoracic nerve arises from the C5, C6 and C7 roots.

Interpretation of haematinic results

122.B   Carcinoma of the rectum
123.D   Extensive jejunal diverticula
124.C   Previous massive small bowel resection
125.A   Previous total gastrectomy
126.E   Chronic haemorrhagic gastritis with acute urinary tract infection

Stems 122 and 126 are examples of microcytic anaemia and are therefore best explained by the two diagnoses associated with chronic blood loss. Iron deficiency is usually characterised by reduced ferritin and raised TIBC. However, if there is an associated brisk inflammatory response, the ferritin may be normal or elevated. The total iron binding capacity is elevated in iron deficiency and is unaffected by sepsis. The macrocytic anaemias in stems 123 and 125 can be attributed to previous total gastrectomy and bacterial overgrowth in jejunal diverticula, both of which cause low serum B_{12}. They can be distinguished from each other by the observation that bacterial overgrowth often results in the synthesis of folate by bacteria. Note that small rises in the serum folate may also accompany B_{12} deficiency without overgrowth. Stem 124 shows an anaemia with normal mean cell volume resulting from a combined deficiency of iron and folate which individually cause microcytosis and macrocytosis respectively.

Treatment of haemostatic disorders

127.E   Platelets, cryoprecipitate and fresh frozen plasma
128.D   Intermediate purity factor VIII concentrate
129.A   Vitamin K and fresh frozen plasma

- This shows the classical clinical and laboratory features of disseminated intravascular coagulation, urgent treatment is required to avert impending haemorrhage. There is prolongation of both the PT and APTT, thrombocytopenia and hypofibrinogenaemia. Treatment is therefore aimed at replacing all clotting factors, platelets and fibrinogen. It is important to also treat the underlying cause.
- This is a commonly encountered presentation of von Willebrand's disease. Haemophilia A shows similar abnormalities in the coagulation screen but is unlikely here because of the gender of the patient, the clinical history and the concordant reduction in both factor VIII and von Willebrand factor. Further investigation is required before surgery to confirm the diagnosis. From the available options, intermediate purity factor VIII is most appropriate as this plasma product contains both factor VIII and von Willebrand factor.
- This provides an example of a patient who has bled due to over-anticoagulation with warfarin and requires emergency surgery. Vitamin K alone will require 24 hours to correct the haemostatic defect and so should be supplemented with fresh frozen plasma which contains the deficient factors II, VII, IX and X.

MRCS CORE INDEX

PASTEST REVISION BOOKS

MRCS Core Modules: Essential Revision Notes   1 901198 36 7
Ed. J Elkabir & A Khadra

MRCS System Modules: Essential Revision Notes   1 901198 41 3
Ed. C Parchment Smith & C Hernon

These new books give a unique presentation of the key elements of all subjects covered in the Core and System Modules syllabus. Unlike conventional textbooks, the essential facts in each subject are presented in note form with special attention given to areas which are often poorly understood. Designed to make learning easier, no candidate should be without these excellent books.

* The definitive guides to revision for the MRCS examination
* Vital facts presented in user-friendly format
* All areas of the syllabus covered in concise note form
* Diagrams, lists, illustrations and bullet points to aid learning
* Essential information highlighted throughout each chapter

MRCS Core Modules: MCQs and EMQs   1 901198 09 X
A Williams, C Chan, T Hennigan & L Barker

MRCS System Modules: MCQs and EMQs   1 901198 10 3
A Williams, C Chan, T Hennigan & L Barker

These two books have been devised to comprehensively cover all aspects of the Core and System Modules necessary for the exam. Extensive explanations are provided for each question and are presented in an easily accessible format.

* Over 300 new MCQs and EMQs covering each of the Modules in its own section
* Correct answers help to identify weak areas of knowledge in time for further study
* Similar in content and level of difficulty to current exam questions
* Expert advice on successful examination technique

214

PASTEST REVISION BOOKS

MRCS Core Modules: Practice Papers   1 901198 45 6
C Chan

MRCS System Modules: Practice Papers   1 901198 46 4
C Chan

Compiled by a team of experienced surgeons, these new books feature five Practice Papers, providing an excellent framework for study and revision for those preparing for the written component of the MRCS exam.

- Five new Practice Papers
- Answers and detailed teaching notes for each question
- Similar in content and level of difficulty to current exam questions
- Expert advice on successful examination technique

To order any of the above titles, please contact PasTest on Freephone:

0800 980 9814

PasTest, FREEPOST, Knutsford, Cheshire, WA16 7BR
Fax: 01565 650264 E-mail: books@pastest.co.uk
or order on-line at www.pastest.co.uk

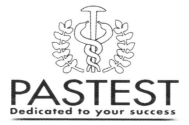

PASTEST
Dedicated to your success

PASTEST REVISION COURSES FOR MRCS

Feeling in need of a helping hand towards success in your exams?

PasTest has over twenty-five years' experience in helping doctors to pass first time, with specially tailored courses to make the most of your valuable revision time.

Over 4000 candidates attend our courses each year at locations throughout the UK. To give you the most up-to-date information and help you to achieve the best results, we constantly update and improve our courses based on feedback from those who attend.

Our course material is continually updated to ensure the best possible revision for the exam. You will receive hundreds of exam-type MCQs and EMQs, with explanations and detailed handouts, and mock exam practice.

- **Two-day MCQ/EMQ Courses**

Intensive revision in either Core Modules or Systems Modules. An opportunity to study over the weekend – ideal if you are unable to take study leave.

- **Three-day MCQ/EMQ Courses**

Following feedback from previous MRCS candidates, we have extended the two-day course to include extra teaching time for the more complex areas.

- **Clinical and Viva Courses**

Run in association with various hospitals, our two-day clinical and viva courses offer small teaching groups to provide you with the best help possible.

HAVE YOU APPLIED FOR FREE PASTEST MEMBERSHIP?

PasTest Membership benefits include access to an exclusive members' area on the PasTest website where you can download free exam material, special members' discounts on courses and books and the most up-to-date revision material throughout your postgraduate study.

For queries on books, courses or benefits of the PasTest Membership scheme, please call our dedicated Customer Services team on **0800 980 9814**. Alternatively, visit our website at **www.pastest.co.uk**.